WHEN HELPING HURTS

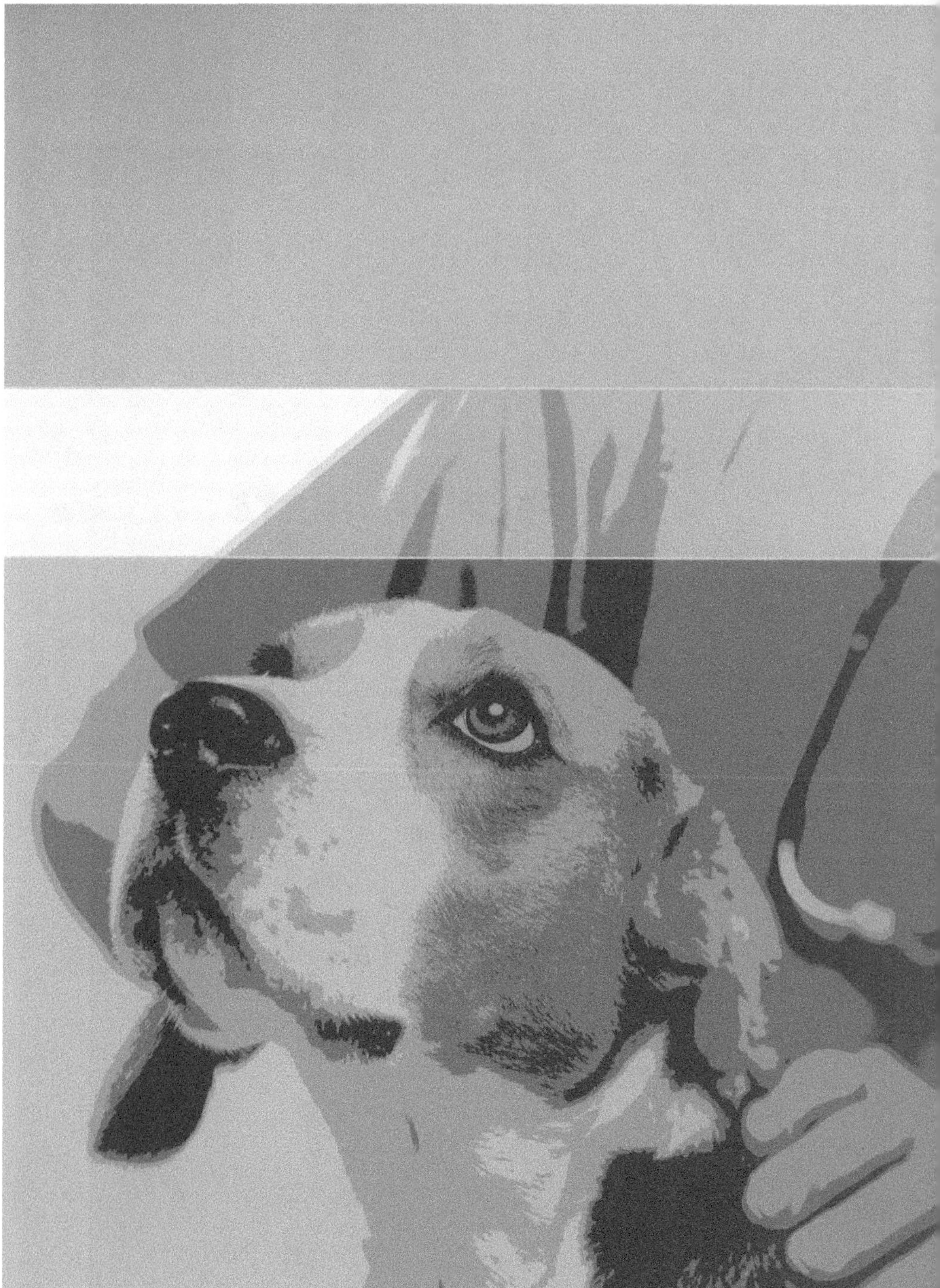

WHEN HELPING HURTS

Compassion Fatigue in the Veterinary Profession

REVISED EDITION

Kathleen Ayl, PsyD

TEXAS A&M UNIVERSITY PRESS
COLLEGE STATION

Revised edition

∞ This paper meets the requirements of ANSI/NISO Z39.48-1992 (Permanence of Paper).
Binding materials have been chosen for durability.
Manufactured in the United States of America.

Library of Congress Cataloging-in-Publication Data

Names: Ayl, Kathleen, 1954– author
Title: When helping hurts: compassion fatigue in the veterinary profession / Kathleen Ayl.
Description: Revised edition. | College Station: Texas A&M University Press, [2026] | Includes bibliographical references and index.
Identifiers: LCCN 2026009333 (print) | LCCN 2026009334 (ebook) | ISBN 9781648434198 paperback | ISBN 9781648434204 ebook
Subjects: LCSH: Veterinarians—Psychology | Veterinary medicine—Social aspects | Pet loss—Psychological aspects | Euthanasia of animals—Psychological aspects | Human-animal relationships | Secondary traumatic stress
Classification: LCC SF740 .A95 2026 (print) | LCC SF740 (ebook)
LC record available at https://lccn.loc.gov/2026009333
LC ebook record available at https://lccn.loc.gov/2026009334

This book complies with the EU General Product Safety Regulation (GPSR) (Regulation (EU) 2023/988). For regulatory inquiries and product safety matters within the EU, contact our authorized representative:

Mare Nostrum Group B.V. | Doelen 72 | 4831 GR Breda | The Netherlands
Email: gpsr@mare-nostrum.co.uk | Website: https://mngbookshop.co.uk/

This publication has undergone a risk assessment and meets applicable safety standards. Traceability identifiers: ISBN, batch number, and publisher contact details are provided for compliance. No hazardous materials or components are included in this product.

Published by Texas A&M University Press
John H. Lindsey Building, Lewis Street | College Station, TX 77843 | www.tamupress.com

Contents

Preface

Even as a small child, I was clear that, as an adult, I wanted to work in a field that helped others improve their quality of life, whether adults or children, pets or any other living beings. All that mattered, by the time I was in the fourth grade, I told myself, was making a difference in the quality of the lives of others, two-legged or four!

What I will never understand is how I got so lucky to have learned from two of the world's greatest beings, Mother Teresa and psychiatrist Dr. Elisabeth Kübler-Ross. An inner and outer knowledge, incredible kindness, and a deep compassion for others surrounded them both.

For the first edition of my award-winning book, *When Helping Hurts: Compassion Fatigue in the Veterinary Profession*, published by the American Animal Hospital Association (AAHA) press in 2013, I won the Bronze Medal in the 2014 Axiom Business Book Awards. AAHA later approached me to write the second edition, which I did. No sooner had it gone to print, however, than the press was shut down by the sudden emergence of the COVID pandemic. AAHA as a publishing house was unable to reopen its doors. Eventually, however, after COVID died down, the good people at Texas A&M University Press gave *When Helping Hurts* another chance, for which I will remain forever grateful.

WHEN HELPING HURTS

PART I

UNDERSTANDING COMPASSION FATIGUE

The Invitation

—ORIAH MOUNTAIN DREAMER

It doesn't interest me what you do for a living.
I want to know what you ache for
and if you dare to dream
of meeting your heart's longing.

It doesn't interest me how old you are.
I want to know if you will risk
looking like a fool for love
for your dream
for the adventure of being alive.

It doesn't interest me what planets are squaring your moon . . .
    I want to know
if you have touched
the centre of your own sorrow if you have been opened
by life's betrayals
or have become shrivelled and closed from fear of further pain.

I want to know
if you can sit with pain mine or your own without moving to hide it
  or fade it
or fix it.

I want to know
if you can be with joy mine or your own
if you can dance with wildness and let the ecstasy fill you
to the tips of your fingers and toes
without cautioning us to be careful
to be realistic
to remember the limitations of being human.

It doesn't interest me
if the story you are telling me is true.
I want to know if you can disappoint another
to be true to yourself.
If you can bear
the accusation of betrayal and not betray your own soul.
If you can be faithless
and therefore trustworthy.

I want to know if you can see Beauty even when it is not pretty
every day.
And if you can source your own life from its presence.

I want to know
if you can live with failure yours and mine
and still stand at the edge of the lake and shout to the silver of
  the full moon,
"Yes."

It doesn't interest me to know where you live
or how much money you have.
I want to know if you can get up after the night of grief and despair
  weary and bruised to the bone and do what needs to be done
to feed the children.

It doesn't interest me who you know
or how you came to be here.
I want to know if you will stand in the centre of the fire
with me
and not shrink back.

It doesn't interest me
where or what or with whom you have studied.
I want to know what sustains you from the inside
when all else falls away.

I want to know
if you can be alone with yourself
and if you truly like the company you keep
in the empty moments.

1

Understanding When Helping Hurts

That which is to give light must also endure burning.

—VICTOR FRANKL

Veterinary care professionals can and do absorb the trauma of the clients and pets with whom they work. Compassion fatigue is the natural result of continual exposure to the suffering of others. Sadly, few veterinary care professionals know how to protect themselves from compassion fatigue. The condition is not unusual; as in many caring professions, it is the very ability to empathize with the suffering of others, and to have compassion to begin with, that leaves the professional caregiver vulnerable to developing it. When we open our hearts to the pain of others, we can be deeply affected.

Defining Compassion Fatigue

One of the world's leading traumatologists, Charles Figley, director of the Tulane University Traumatology Institute, described compassion fatigue as a type of "secondary stress disorder." He suggested that "the display of symptoms is the natural consequence of stress resulting from caring and helping traumatized or suffering people or animals" (Figley 1995). Charles Figley and Robert Roop wrote that compassion fatigue was a "deep awareness of the suffering of another coupled with the wish to relieve it." They stated it was "a kind of focused, action-oriented empathy" (Figley and Roop 2006, 10–11).

Many researchers have described how working with trauma can compromise our ego resources—that is, our ability to manage interpersonal relationships and set appropriate relationship boundaries. This ego-resource depletion can make it less likely that we will be able to decide on our own best interest, and, according to psychologists Karen W. Saakvitne and Laurie Anne Pearlman (1996), professional errors in setting boundaries and using judgment will be more likely. For this reason, I advise all my compassion-fatigued professionals to avoid making any major decisions for a while, if possible. The likelihood of making a decision we will later regret is much higher when such overwhelming emotions are present.

Compassion fatigue—or, as it has also been called, vicarious traumatization or secondary trauma—was first diagnosed in the medical field in the 1950s. Since that time, a wealth of new research has shed light on the condition. This book provides you with the latest information on compassion fatigue to help you apply it to your own situation and the people around you who may be experiencing it. Suppose you are a manager or a veterinary hospital owner. In that case, you will learn how to prevent your employees from spiraling into compassion fatigue and what to do when you see its effects.

What does compassion fatigue look like? Compassion fatigue affects different people in different ways, but it can follow similar patterns. Sheila, for example, was a young, highly dedicated veterinarian when I first met her twelve years ago. She had a positive outlook, was excited about her profession, and had a vibrant and engaging personality. But when I recently reconnected with her, I found that she had become angry, lonely, and cynical. She was overwhelmed by her workload, her difficult clients, and the ongoing losses she faced. She reported finding herself often uncharacteristically angry or frustrated by clients, staff, or even the checkout woman at the grocery store. Sheila realized something was wrong but didn't know how to fix it. So she threw herself more and more into her profession, trying to get things together while being pulled down even further into compassion fatigue.

Compassion itself is a unique emotion. It is a little like sympathy, but it does not mean feeling sorry for someone else, as many might assume (see textbox "What Is Compassion?"). Compassion for others, like sympathy—and also like another closely related emotion, empathy—comes from the heart, but it specifically denotes being present in an energetic way for someone who has been traumatized or is suffering. In veterinary care, that "someone" includes not just people (clients) but also animals (patients). When you have compassion, you do not just "feel" something; you also "do" something to help.

What Is Compassion?

Compassion, empathy, and sympathy are closely related terms. In everyday conversation, they may often be interchangeable. However, when discussing compassion fatigue, we want to be precise about definitions. To understand how a person can spiral into compassion fatigue, we must begin by understanding what compassion is. The following basic definitions of these three terms will help lay the foundation for an understanding of compassion fatigue.

Sympathy: Similarity or agreement between two or more individuals relating to a viewpoint or emotional response. The verb "to sympathize" means to experience this similarity of views or emotions. For example, "I sympathize with his views, as I have come to the same conclusions myself."

Empathy: The capacity to see things from another's point of view and feel what that person is feeling. The verb "to empathize" means to experience this capacity. For example, "I empathized with him—I could feel the pain myself when he described his predicament."

Compassion: A heartfelt understanding of the difficult situation of another to the point that one is moved to take action of some sort. For example, "The veterinarian had such compassion for the animal that she worked through the night to save his life."

Compassion focuses on those empathetic or sympathetic feelings and puts them into action.

Compassion fatigue is a very real problem in veterinary medicine—and in any profession in which caregivers face repeated, long-term exposure to the suffering and loss of others. The tasks in these professions often require superhuman physical and emotional strength and a seemingly endless supply of compassion. With the continual demands placed on the veterinary professional's time and energy and the huge amount of ongoing, day-to-day stress, it's no wonder that compassion fatigue can set in. Empathy and compassion are necessary qualities for anyone working in veterinary care. They allow the individual to connect with clients, to care about the animals, and to provide the best possible care. But these emotions, if not checked, can also backfire.

A person who is experiencing compassion fatigue is devastated by the repeated exposure to the pain and trauma of others, which leaves the caregiver feeling overwhelmed, angry, exhausted, and, ultimately, unable to care about anything. When left unaddressed, the condition can lead to career dissatisfaction, high employee turnover rates, and even substance abuse or suicide. The veterinary field is becoming increasingly aware of the profound cumulative effect that witnessing suffering and pain can have on veterinary professionals. And yet many people who are experiencing it don't realize they are suffering from compassion fatigue. In any discussion of compassion fatigue, it must be distinguished from other, similar terms, such as secondary traumatic stress, vicarious trauma, grief, and even stress and burnout (see textbox "Making Distinctions"). Figley and Roop wrote, "Conceptually, researchers have attempted to differentiate compassion fatigue from burnout, vicarious trauma, and general psychological distress, but the terms have remained imprecise" (2006, 25). However, it is possible to make general distinctions.

First, let's look at stress and burnout in relation to compassion fatigue.

Compassion fatigue involves emotional, physical, mental, social, and spiritual changes resulting from engaging empathetically with animals and people who have been traumatized or are experiencing a traumatic event. Patricia Smith, the founder of the Compassion Fatigue Awareness Project (CFAP), described it as the result of "giving care to people or animals in pain or who are suffering" (2009). She suggests that we should "think of stress as 'too much'—too much work, too many hours, too many expectations," and of burnout "as 'not enough'; that is, feelings of depletion, emptiness, apathy, and lack of motivation." As she goes on to explain, "Compassion fatigue is neither; it is the emotional stress that arises when a caregiver takes on the pain and suffering of others and claims it as his or her own. Unfortunately, by the time a caregiver recognizes the symptoms of compassion fatigue, chances are good that he or she also is suffering from both traumatic stress and burnout."

Both stress and burnout can result from various factors unrelated to compassion per se (for example, too many demands on your time, difficult relationships, or chronic illness). They can, in fact, occur in fields in which there is little interaction with others (for example, accounting). Whereas some forms of stress and burnout might be alleviated by a week off in Hawaii, compassion fatigue requires more attention if recovery is to occur. Compassion fatigue must be addressed and dealt with continually and proactively.

Stress is the natural result of excessive pressures in your life, but what is felt to be "excessive" is completely subjective. According to the American Institute of Stress, Hans Selye, an endocrinologist, first defined the word "stress" in its current usage in 1936. He said it was "the nonspecific response of the body to any demand for change."

Making Distinctions

With all the terms related to compassion fatigue swirling around in your head, sometimes it isn't easy to keep them straight. Here are brief definitions of each. While reading later sections of the book, you may wish to return to these definitions to review them, but do read through them now as well. It is important not to blur these distinctions as you attempt to identify and cope with compassion fatigue.

Burnout: A condition that occurs when, in responding to excessive stresses and demands, you demand too much of yourself, eventually becoming overwhelmed, exhausted, apathetic, and negative.

Compassion fatigue: Acute emotional pain accompanied by physical, spiritual, and mental exhaustion that stems from caregiving. Working continually with the suffering of others while not taking care of your own needs leads to an unbalanced and unhealthy lifestyle. It has been likened to a combination of burnout and secondary traumatic stress.

Grief: A normal response to loss. It is a period of intensely painful emotions that begins with the loss of a loved one. Intense grief can dominate your entire life.

Post-traumatic stress disorder: An anxiety disorder that occurs after you experience or observe a traumatic event involving significant injury, death, or the threat thereof.

Secondary traumatic stress: A component of compassion fatigue that involves work-related, secondary exposure to extremely stressful events. The symptoms of secondary traumatic stress echo those of the patient and are usually rapid in onset and associated with a particular event.

Stress: The emotional, mental, and/or physical strain that results from too many pressures and demands in your life, typically from external sources. Stress can contribute to burnout and compassion fatigue.

Vicarious trauma: The cumulative negative effect of experiencing the trauma of others, to the extent that it can result in dissociation from both professional and personal relationships, as well as intrusive images and nightmares, despair, and resignation.

Burnout is more debilitating than stress. According to the Wholistic Stress Control Institute, it is "a condition that evolves slowly over a period of prolonged stress." The institute's website describes burnout as a "wearing down and wearing out of energy" by "excessive demands which may be self-imposed by families, jobs, friends, value systems, or society, which depletes one's energy, coping mechanisms, and internal resources." It is also "accompanied by an overload of stress, which eventually impacts one's motivation, attitudes, and behaviors."

Compassion fatigue is not the same as burnout. Burnout is associated with excessive demands and stressors that are involved in the type of work you do. It is a cumulative process that can often be remedied by a vacation from work. Not so with compassion fatigue, which is complete physical and spiritual exhaustion accompanied by acute emotional pain, all of which stems from working as a caregiver and dealing continually with the suffering of others while not taking good enough care of your own needs.

Post-traumatic stress disorder (PTSD), unlike stress and burnout, is not a result of everyday situations; it is a response to trauma. From the fifth edition of the *Diagnostic and Statistical Manual of Mental Disorders* (DSM-5), we learn that PTSD is a reaction that lasts more than a month, causes significant distress, and is caused by being directly exposed to either real or threatened death, sexual violence, or serious injury. It can occur through learning that a loved one was threatened by a severe accident; through violence; through witnessing a traumatic event involving another being; or through listening firsthand to graphic details, as with the descriptions relayed to veterinary professionals, therapists, first responders, or police officers following a traumatic event. For a diagnosis of PTSD to be made, the trauma response must also include at least one of the following intrusion-associated symptoms: distressing and recurrent thoughts of the event; recurrent or distressing dreams about the traumatic incident; physiological reactions in response to cues that resemble an aspect of the trauma; dissociative reactions such as flashbacks and intense psychological distress when exposed to something that symbolizes an aspect of the trauma. There must also be evidence of persistent avoidance of stimuli associated with the incident by either seeking to avoid or avoiding distressing thoughts and memories or feelings of the trauma, or avoiding all reminders of the traumatic event. There can also be negative changes in thoughts and moods associated with the trauma and changes in arousal and reactivity associated with the trauma.

In my opinion, primary and secondary PTSD and compassion fatigue are similar in at least one way: they involve the restriction of feelings. You try to ignore your feelings or become numb to them. Compassion fatigue is what damages veterinary professionals the most. It is understandable to try to protect yourself by not feeling the pain. But the more you ignore your feelings—by running from them or trying to bury them in an effort not to feel them—the more power you give them.

The distinctions between workplace stress, burnout, post-traumatic stress, and compassion fatigue are fairly clear, but secondary traumatic stress and vicarious trauma are more closely connected concepts. Many experts believe compassion fatigue is the same as secondary traumatic stress. Drs. Laura Simpson and Donna Starkey emphasized the importance of looking at the effects that working with traumatized clients can have on the psychological well-being of their caretakers. "These ancillary effects," they wrote, "frequently experienced by those not directly traumatized, are often defined as secondary trauma or compassion fatigue" (Simpson and Starkey 2006). Recent work has shown that secondary traumatic stress is part of compassion fatigue, which crystallizes around fear and echoes the traumatic experiences of the person being helped (Stamm 2010; Huggard, Stamm, and Pearlman 2013). The initial signs of a 2022 study suggest that an online program designed to help informal caregivers with compassion fatigue, burnout, and secondary traumatic stress could be a practical way to support their mental well-being (Koller, Abel, and Milton 2022). Both compassion fatigue and secondary trauma are related to the caretaking role, whereby we help people or animals that are suffering. The symptoms are only intensified when veterinary professionals try to bury their feelings in an effort to carry on. As mentioned above, the notion that you can just ignore these feelings is a common misconception, and we explore this further later in the book. For now, know that nothing will further the progression of compassion fatigue faster than not dealing with it.

In a very informative article, Rachel Rauvola, Dulce Vega, and Kristi Lavigne (2019) offer a qualitative review summarizing the literature published over the last decade that pertains to work-related, empathy-based stress, such as compassion fatigue and secondary traumatic stress. Life coach and former veterinarian Dr. Jeni Waeltz refers to secondary traumatic stress as the largely overlooked and misunderstood side of compassion fatigue (2019). Beth Stamm (2010) states that for most, "compassion fatigue is viewed as a multidimensional construct composed of two dimensions, burnout and secondary traumatic stress. Unlike burnout, which is a cumulative process, secondary traumatic stress is acute." The emotional duress resulting from secondary traumatic stress happens without being directly involved with the traumatic experience, including not having to witness it. Its symptoms are similar to those of PTSD, and its etiology is listening firsthand to the distressing details of the traumatic experiences of another person.

Grief, in contrast, is a primary trauma rather than a secondary one. Grief is a major factor in dissatisfaction in veterinary hospital settings because of the constant exposure to death. In some important ways, the effects of recurring grief are indistinguishable from the effects of compassion fatigue and may also contribute to compassion fatigue. Later, when we discuss the human-animal bond, grief will be an integral part of that discussion. Many self-care strategies for dealing with compassion fatigue are also effective at combating the effects of recurring grief.

Veterinary care professionals spend day after day in close proximity to vulnerable people and pets in need of help. More often than not, veterinary team members also know a great deal about the private lives and challenges of their clients and their families. At a moment's notice, they could rattle off a client's relevant personal history (e.g., "five months ago, she unfortunately lost her husband of thirty-six years"), primary personal relationships (e.g., "he does have one son, but I believe he lives in Tennessee, and there is no one else left here in California"), and the relevant support system (e.g., "there appears to be no friends or family, but she did mention that she goes to church every Sunday"). This is all extremely important information, and having it on hand helps you be the best veterinary team member you can be. The fact that veterinary care providers have so much information memorized also shows just how strong the human element is in veterinary practice. Your clients become a part of your life as a veterinary professional.

Many factors contribute to compassion fatigue. Physical and emotional exhaustion, ongoing exposure to the trauma of others, problematic clients or coworkers, problems separating your personal life from your career, and poor communication in the work environment can all play a role.

The Need for Safeguards

As much as veterinary caregivers care about their clients, they also must safeguard themselves. Anna, a veterinary professional with whom I have had the pleasure of working, couldn't understand why she was uncharacteristically angry all the time. "It's just not me," she said. "I snap at people all the time: my friends, family, coworkers, and people I don't even know! I don't recognize myself anymore."

Anna, like Sheila, described earlier, and most of the other veterinary professionals with whom I have spoken, initially felt a strong pull to help alleviate animal suffering and illness. But many of these same people have become disillusioned. They are disappointed by the difference between what their dream was and the reality of the work that confronts them daily. Sadly, they have lost the joy that they once felt in practicing veterinary medicine. Many have described how a sense of emptiness, numbness, or disconnection has taken its place.

It is unknown how prevalent compassion fatigue is in veterinary medicine; more research is needed. However, veterinary researchers have begun to identify some of the factors that put veterinary employees at risk. For example, in "The Compassion Satisfaction and Fatigue Survey," conducted in 2003–04, the Humane Society of the United States asked veterinarians, veterinary technicians, and veterinary assistants, along with front-office staff and management, about their jobs to help identify the highest stressors in the profession. The survey also measured job satisfaction. The survey results were as follows:

- Veterinarians' highest stressors were difficult or noncompliant clients, lack of time, and having to discuss or dispute their fees. Their highest sources of satisfaction were being able to help animals, clients who appreciated their services and were thankful, and the feeling of working together as a team.
- For veterinary technicians and veterinary assistants, the number one stressor was having to deal with difficult clients, followed by difficulties with coworkers and lack of time. Their highest source of satisfaction also came from being able to help the animals; the next highest was working together as a team and having appreciative clients.
- For front-office professionals and management, the number one stressor was, again, difficult or noncompliant clients. Demanding time schedules and disputes over fees or billing were second and third, respectively. Their primary sources of satisfaction were clients who were appreciative and thankful, being able to have contact with animals daily, and being a part of helping animals.

Veterinary professionals are under pressure to meet the needs of their patients as well as the expectations of their clients. Additionally, some of those clients are highly demanding, whereas others may need to be more realistic. Doing far more for far less and taking on the stress and strain of someone else's problems and difficulties can sometimes seem intolerable. Continual exposure to trauma and grief is an ongoing challenge in the veterinary profession. When those inherent challenges are coupled with financial pressures (such as clients sometimes not being able to afford treatment or not having a retirement plan), it's no wonder that so many veterinary care providers are succumbing to the symptoms of compassion fatigue.

Most veterinary professionals know that if they had chosen to go into human medicine, they would be making far more money and have full benefits. Yet they chose to turn down that option and go into veterinary care because of their commitment to the animals. They didn't expect the stress they would feel from witnessing their patients' pain and often their clients' grief. When they do experience these things, they may prefer feeling numb to the gut-wrenching pain that can result from caring too much. As Simon and Garfunkel put it so well in the lyrics of their brilliant song "I Am a Rock," being numb keeps a person from feeling too much pain or sorrow. However, by shutting down their feelings in an attempt to avoid feeling the pain, veterinary care professionals can find that they also miss out on some of the joy and other positive feelings life brings. They may stop responding to life and those with whom they have relationships in open and honest ways. Nothing could be more detrimental emotionally for the veterinary care professional or the client.

It is clear that veterinary team members who are affected by compassion fatigue may not be performing at their best on the job. Compassion fatigue can rob you of the ability to concentrate, causing a decrease in job performance while increasing the number of mistakes a team member makes. Compassion fatigue is associated with increased absences from work, a heightened risk of substance abuse, and all sorts of relationship problems both at home and in the workplace.

Not being honest or true to yourself causes your self-esteem to plummet, and it harms grieving clients. Most pet owners begin grieving the moment they suspect or hear a terminal diagnosis. They feel vulnerable, and as a result, they often become hypervigilant. Consciously or subconsciously, they attempt to seek out people with whom they feel safe and places that are comforting. If veterinary professionals are not knowledgeable about their own feelings, clients will not find the sense of safety they seek. Consequently, clients will not be amenable to the support and kindness the caregivers hope to extend.

Preventing compassion fatigue is possible, but only if veterinary team members are vigilant about taking care of themselves. In a study of the relationship between self-care, compassion satisfaction, compassion fatigue, and burnout, researchers found that when people experiencing low levels of burnout and compassion fatigue used self-care strategies, they had higher levels of compassion satisfaction (Alkema, Linton, and Davies 2008). In short, if a veterinary caregiver experiences continual, direct contact with animals and people who are traumatized while engaging empathetically with them, and fails to practice ongoing self-care, the caregiver is at a high risk of developing compassion fatigue. Veterinary care puts enormous physical and emotional demands on veterinary professionals, and as a result, veterinary professionals are logically predisposed to compassion fatigue. To remain compassionate without being consumed by the pain and trauma of others, caregivers must maintain their boundaries through the ongoing practice of self-awareness and self-care.

This book is for you, the veterinary care professional. If your stress and fatigue levels are low, it will help you design a self-care program to prevent compassion fatigue from developing further. If you are suffering from a greater degree of compassion fatigue, it will help you reestablish and reaffirm your desire and ability to support yourself and others through trauma and loss or the impending loss of loved ones. It is meant for anyone employed in the veterinary care profession. For if you work with those who are traumatized, you are at high risk of developing compassion fatigue. This book will provide you with the resources you will need to recognize, address, and prevent compassion fatigue. It is designed to spark personal renewal and provide you with a way to help other team members. You will be offered information, advice, and exercises regarding emotionally difficult situations that result from the trauma, loss, or potential loss of a patient or other traumas experienced by you, your coworkers, and your clients.

I hope that this book will help you to

- Understand and be aware of the symptoms of compassion fatigue.
- Assess your level of sensitivity as an individual through self-assessment evaluations.
- Assess your personal compassion fatigue and your current level of self-care through self-assessment evaluations.
- Prevent and heal the stress and trauma inherent in caring for others.
- Learn helpful and healing exercises you can do to care for yourself while you are caring for others.
- Build your resiliency and develop ways of maintaining your balance.
- Learn ways to manage anger and frustration without damaging relationships.

- Learn how to set personal boundaries and honor yourself enough to follow them.
- Learn emotional and physical relaxation techniques.
- Discover the importance of building a support system.
- Discover (or rediscover) the sense of meaning and reward you get from your work.
- Understand ways of expressing your inner self through the creative arts.
- Face and heal any personal issues you have that may compel you to take on more than you should.
- Help coworkers or employees learn to recognize the symptoms of compassion fatigue and engage actively in prevention, to rediscover their sense of joy in the field of veterinary practice, and to get help when needed.

Remember, higher stress levels will equal lower levels of functioning in both your professional tasks and your personal life. The benefits of understanding and dealing appropriately with compassion fatigue go well beyond the basic benefit of finding relief. Once you have rediscovered the joy of helping, you will benefit professionally and personally in many ways you cannot now imagine—and so will your family and friends, coworkers, clients, and patients.

We have been making distinctions in this chapter. However, in real life, these distinctions will not seem so clear. Your own grief for a dying pet will affect you at the same time that you are feeling overwhelmed by compassion for a client. You may be experiencing PTSD and compassion fatigue simultaneously, not to mention that everyday stress or burnout will make it more difficult for you to handle your distress. Now that you know the definitions of each term, you may see some of the threads of each in how you feel. This book will help, no matter how many of the terms we've discussed apply to your situation.

For the Trainer

After reading chapter 1, either on your own or as a group, discuss the following:

1. How would you compare and contrast stress, burnout, grief, post-traumatic stress and/or secondary traumatic stress, and compassion fatigue based on your experience or observations?

2. What do you think are some of the factors contributing to compassion fatigue?
3. How prevalent do you think compassion fatigue is in veterinary practice, based on your own observations?
4. If you suspected that you or a coworker were suffering from compassion fatigue, would you know what to do? Would you like to know what to do?

2

Inner and Outer Factors Leading to Compassion Fatigue

I can be changed by what happens to me. But I refuse to be reduced by it.

—MAYA ANGELOU

Most veterinary professionals come into the field with a strong sense of calling and a desire to serve pets and their people. Once these professionals have completed their training and entered the veterinary practice setting, they confront some of life's most difficult situations. They often find that their training did not fully equip them to cope with the suffering they witness daily.

Yes, practicing veterinary medicine can be very rewarding. But it also takes an enormous toll financially, spiritually, mentally, and physically. The toll is exacted on every team member—not just veterinarians. Technicians, front-desk staff, and others are equally affected because all practice employees are subject to many of the same risks and are often affected by the same causes of compassion fatigue.

In later chapters, you will learn self-care strategies to help you thrive in veterinary practice. But first, in this chapter, we explore the many causes of compassion fatigue. Increasing your awareness of the causes is the first step toward prevention and recovery. As it turns out, both internal and external factors contribute to compassion fatigue, and these combine in different ways for different people. Although we examine them one by one, keep in mind that how they add up and accumulate, especially over time, enhances the risk of developing compassion fatigue.

Case Study | Karen

Karen, a highly skilled veterinary technician from a small specialty practice, had worked in the field for seven years. She told me she had wanted to work in the veterinary field her entire life because of her great love for animals. "I thought I came into the veterinary field for all the right reasons," she said. "I used to love to see the patients and the clients. But I am finding that the longer I am in the field, the more difficult it is for me to care. I don't know what happened to the joy I once had in my profession. My pay is certainly not enough to compensate for all this job takes from me. By the time I go home, I feel like I have nothing left for my family, much less myself. I don't think I can do this anymore."

Internal Factors

Human beings are physiologically wired to take on the emotions and pain of others. Did you ever notice that when people interact closely over time, they begin to take on one another's postures and facial expressions? Most people smile responsively to someone who is smiling at them. An upbeat attitude is typically met with an upbeat attitude. Why? Because it is not only the expression but also the feeling that gets transmitted. Most people with a sense of social awareness have noticed this. Amazingly, the same principle holds true for emotions we think of as being more negative. When facial expressions associated with sadness, anger, or fear are copied, the feelings, too, can be transmitted.

In this way, the very ability to experience emotion and pick up on the emotional cues of others is the first internal factor in compassion fatigue. Also at work are personality type, lack of assertiveness, perfectionism, and sensitivity to suffering. Many other factors can put a person at risk of developing compassion fatigue. Some of these have to do with unique circumstances, and we will not have time to explore each one in depth. (However, I list some of them at the end of this section.) Here, we look briefly at each of the primary internal factors in compassion fatigue.

Ability to Experience Emotion

The body is an important component in how we experience emotion. That's because the emotions we experience daily correspond to brain activity, which in turn is affected by the external stimuli we experience. Emotions can then influence our behavior.

For example, empathetic reactions can be elicited by any one of the five senses. Have you ever felt physical pain when you witnessed someone falling and scraping her knee? This ability to mimic the activity of someone else's brain cells occurs through mirror neurons, which allow us to activate the same neurons within our own brains by observing an action as by performing it. Mirror neurons are involved in a large number of human interactions.

This "mirroring" has been demonstrated in experiments by neuroscientists. For example, in one study, pain-sensitive brain neurons were activated not only in subjects whose fingers were pricked with needles but also in other subjects who had only observed the other subjects having their fingers pricked. The neurons created an empathetic connection between the observers and those who were experiencing the pain (Hutchison et al. 1999).

When the emotions we experience are traumatic, they can have a dramatic effect on our behavior. The importance of the stimulus that elicits the emotion is a central factor in determining our behavior and its impact on our lives and the lives of others. Studies with titles such as "The Key Role of the Amygdala in Stress" (Andolina and Borreca 2017); "'It's All in the Eyes': The Role of the Amygdala in the Experience and Perception of Fear" (Massachusetts General Hospital 2018); and "Impaired Left Amygdala Resting State Functional Connectivity in Subthreshold Depression Individuals" (Peng et al. 2020) show that an important limbic structure, the amygdala, is largely responsible for evaluating the emotional significance of the various stimuli a person encounters. The prefrontal and temporal cortical areas share reciprocal connections, and both continually project to other limbic structures.

Therefore, the cortex is very much involved in an emotional response to something you observe or encounter. The loss of a loved one, the loss of something cherished, or even the fear of such loss elicits sadness and a sense of devastation. Because of mirror neurons, when you regularly interact with clients who are experiencing these emotions, you will take on these emotions to some degree. The bottom line is that these emotions are very real. When we talk about emotions, they are not amorphous and "touchy-feely." Something is going on in the brain as you experience them. There is a reason you feel sad when your clients feel sad and cheer right alongside them when their pets recover. Over time, if the negatives are not balanced by positives and mitigated by self-care strategies, they can impact you and may cause compassion fatigue.

Personality Types

Veterinarians and other veterinary team members may be especially prone to compassion fatigue because of the personality determinants that drew them to the profession to begin with. Some experts believe compassion fatigue stems from the need to "rescue" or protect others. Veterinary professionals often exhibit these traits. It isn't money that draws them into the field. They love animals and want to help them; they have a strong sense of calling.

Personality tests can help pinpoint common traits among different professions. Perhaps the best known of these is the Myers-Briggs Type Indicator (MBTI), developed in 1943 by Isabel Briggs Myers and Katharine Briggs (see www.myersbriggs.org/my-mbti-personality-type/mbti-basics/). The MBTI is based on the work of psychiatrist Carl Jung. Jung identified various psychological types and believed that most behavior is consistent and orderly, and therefore somewhat predictable.

Psychologist David Keirsey has created a similar assessment tool called the Jung Typology Test (see www.humanmetrics.com/personality). This test takes less than fifteen minutes to complete. One personality type Keirsey identifies is the "Guardian Protector," who, according to Keirsey, wants to be of service to others and finds great fulfillment in helping those in need. According to Keirsey's website (keirsey.com), Guardian Protectors have a "primary interest in the safety and security of those they care about—their family, their circle of friends, their students, their patients, their boss, their fellow workers, or their employees." The Guardian Protector is a good example of the type of person who may be drawn to veterinary caregiving and who may have a level of compassion for others that could make the development of compassion fatigue more likely. Dozens of other tests like Keirsey's attempt to identify personality traits and relate them to a person's primary desires and goals.

Companion-animal care has become the focus of what was once a male-dominated, agriculturally based industry. More women are entering the profession, and, as in most other medical practices, veterinary medicine is also seeing a shift to a greater emphasis on good communication skills.

In the past, veterinary students tended to be reliable, conscientious, determined, and logical in their communication. They also tended to be task oriented. In recent years, however, the more "feeling" types of personalities, rather than the more "thinking" types, have been entering the field in increasing numbers. This is true regardless of gender.

The American Veterinary Medical Association (AVMA 2020b) noted that besides good science and math skills and the desire to help animals, those applying to veterinary school should also have the prospective school's prerequisites as well as proven leadership abilities, good communication skills, and positive letters of recommendation, especially from former and current employers. With veterinary schools now placing more emphasis on "people skills," entrants to the field may, in general, tend to be more compassionate and empathetic than their predecessors, which also means that they may be more susceptible to compassion fatigue.

Of course, these are broad trends; clearly, there have always been compassionate individuals entering the field, and many new veterinarians today are still task oriented. Knowing your personality type perhaps gives you a better understanding of yourself and how you work. It also helps you become aware of the risks you will face as you act on your natural impulses to help others. Ultimately, you can learn to help yourself, your clients, your patients, and your staff.

Lack of Assertiveness

In general, it has been said that a high percentage of veterinary professionals appear to have an inherent difficulty with saying no to others. Somewhere along the line, they began believing that the needs of others took precedence over their own. They struggle with the issue of boundaries regarding their time, energy, and health. They are often described as good-hearted or caring, but they tend to jump to say yes before they consider the personal costs it will entail. It's often as if saying "I can't do that" doesn't even occur to them.

Maintaining personal boundaries, including saying no, may sound easy to some, but it can be extremely difficult for veterinary caregivers. We must learn how to make healthy decisions that are good for ourselves and others. This is a huge challenge for caregivers of all types. To continue doing what we do, we must learn to recognize and respect our own limits.

If we do not recognize our limits, we become entrenched in them. If you continually give to others without a break, you set yourself up for compassion fatigue. You can empower yourself by not allowing yourself to become overwhelmed. When you take good care of yourself, everyone wins. "Assertiveness is the ability to express one's feelings and assert one's rights while respecting the feelings and rights of others," according to stress management guide Elizabeth Scott. "Assertive communication," she wrote, "is appropriately direct, open, and honest, and clarifies one's needs to the other person. Assertiveness comes naturally to some but is a skill that can be learned. People who have mastered the skill of assertiveness are able to greatly reduce the level of interpersonal conflict in their lives, thereby reducing a major source of stress" (Scott 2023).

Scott was not writing about compassion fatigue per se but about stress in general. However, the lack of assertiveness does play a significant role in the development of compassion fatigue because compassion fatigue so often comes about insidiously over time by the accumulation of emotional responses. If caregivers cannot easily say no, they are much more likely to continually take on more than they can handle without a break, absorbing more and more distressing emotions without having a chance to regroup and recover. Assertiveness training is a valuable tool that can and should be taught to all veterinary care professionals.

Perfectionism

Most veterinary care professionals have unusually high expectations of themselves and commonly tie their sense of self or their personal identity to their profession. According to equine journalist Candy Lawrence in an article on suicides among veterinary professionals, perfectionism is a common trait in veterinary caregivers. They are typically "intent on improving themselves and dedicated to putting forth a 180% effort," and "as a whole, they are deeply committed to the welfare of their patients and clients." However, "when they fail to heal, when they fail to prolong the quality of life, this is often perceived as an internalized, magnified and personal defeat. High levels of self-criticism are often associated with high levels of depression. The mental, spiritual and emotional balance necessary in the field of veterinary medicine is often one of the most difficult if not elusive traits to maintain" (Lawrence 2009).

According to veterinary researcher David Bartram, in an article dealing with the high suicide rate among veterinarians in the United Kingdom, "The stress begins while they're still in training. Typically, entrance to veterinary schools is limited to high achievers, whose personality traits may include neurosis, conscientiousness and perfectionism" (as cited in Watkins 2010).

When perfectionism is added to a situation in which the professional caregiver identifies strongly with the losses of others and becomes overinvolved with patients and clients, this can create insurmountable stress.

Perfectionists may be compassionate to everyone except themselves. When losses occur, veterinary caregivers who are also perfectionists may blame themselves, fretting over what they could have done differently to produce a better outcome. When this occurs repeatedly, it is no wonder that compassion fatigue is the result. Perfectionism is exhausting because there is rarely perfection in life. No matter how well you have done, if you are a perfectionist, you will feel that you should have or could have done a little bit

Are You a Perfectionist?

If you are the type of person who tends to be hard on yourself, you will almost assuredly propel yourself toward compassion fatigue faster than your colleagues. Many veterinary professionals are, by nature, very hard on themselves without realizing it. Ask yourself the following questions to determine whether you fall into this category:

- Are you intolerant of things you do not like about yourself?
- Do you continually judge yourself?
- Do you often feel inadequate?
- Do you tend to ruminate on the things you feel you could have done better?
- Do you expect things to go badly?
- Do you feel as though other people are generally happier than you are?

If you said yes to more than two of these questions, you are struggling with having compassion for yourself. If that is so, try to accept yourself without judgment. Be more compassionate and kinder toward yourself when you are hurting, overwhelmed, or afraid. Try to keep in mind that everyone feels inadequate from time to time. You are not identified by your failings but by your successes. Seek out your balance and remember the times when you felt successful. In later chapters, we will look into how to follow this advice.

better. Constantly seeking perfection will wear you down (see textbox "Are You a Perfectionist?").

Sensitivity to Suffering

Traumatologist Eric Gentry believes that those attracted to a caregiving occupation already suffer from compassion fatigue (as cited in Compassion Fatigue Awareness Project 2010). He suggests that the motive for such work is often a strong identification with the suffering or helplessness of others who have been traumatized. Most people in these occupations, he suggests, at some point interpreted the importance of putting the needs of others ahead of their own as paramount. The idea of proactive self-care is commonly nonexistent in a highly sensitive caregiver's life or thought processes.

Elaine N. Aron, in her groundbreaking book *The Highly Sensitive Person* (2020), defined and explained the issues and challenges faced by highly

Are You Highly Sensitive? A Self-Test

The following self-test was created by Elaine N. Aron and appears in her book *The Highly Sensitive Person*. Aron instructs the reader to "answer each question according to the way you feel. Answer true if it is at least somewhat true for you. Answer false if it is not very true or not at all true for you."

I am aware of the subtleties in my environment.	T	F
Other people's moods affect me.	T	F
I tend to be very sensitive to pain.	T	F
I find myself needing to withdraw during busy days, into bed, a darkened room, or any place where I can have some privacy and relief from stimulation.	T	F
I am particularly sensitive to the effects of caffeine.	T	F
I am easily overwhelmed by things like bright lights, strong smells, coarse fabrics, or sirens close by.	T	F
I have a rich, complex inner life.	T	F
I am made uncomfortable by loud noises.	T	F
I am deeply moved by the arts or music.	T	F
I am conscientious.	T	F
I startle easily.	T	F
I get rattled when I have a lot to do in a short amount of time.	T	F
When people are uncomfortable in a physical environment, I tend to know what needs to be done to make it more comfortable (like changing the lighting or the seating).	T	F
I am annoyed when people try to get me to do too many things at once.	T	F

I try hard to avoid making mistakes or forgetting things.	T	F
I make it a point to avoid violent movies and TV shows.	T	F
I become unpleasantly aroused when a lot is going on around me.	T	F
Being very hungry creates a strong reaction in me, disrupting my concentration or mood.	T	F
Changes in my life shake me up.	T	F
I notice and enjoy delicate or fine scents, tastes, sounds, works, or art.	T	F
I make it a high priority to arrange my life to avoid upsetting or overwhelming situations.	T	F
When I must compete or be observed while performing a task, I become so nervous or shaky that I do much worse than I would otherwise.	T	F
When I was a child, my parents or teachers seemed to see me as sensitive or shy.	T	F

Scoring: Aron says: "If you answered true to twelve or more questions, you're probably highly sensitive. But frankly, no psychological test is so accurate that you should base your life on it. If only one or two questions are true of you, but they are extremely true, you might also be justified in calling yourself highly sensitive."

sensitive persons, or HSPs. She described HSPs as having very sensitive nervous systems, a trait that she believes affects one out of every five people. Researchers call this trait sensory-processing sensitivity, and Aron uses the terms interchangeably. She created a self-test to measure sensitivity levels (see textbox "Are You Highly Sensitive?"). Scoring information helps you determine your placement on the scale.

Being highly sensitive can have its advantages. For example, HSPs are more acutely aware of the subtleties in their surroundings than non-HSPs. However, being hypersensitive can also predispose HSPs to compassion fatigue. Because of their acute awareness, HSPs can become overwhelmed in highly stimulating environments, and veterinary hospitals certainly qualify as highly stimulating.

As mentioned in the introduction to this section, it would be impossible to discuss all the internal factors contributing to compassion fatigue, especially because many are unique to an individual's past experience or natural tendencies. For example, if previous unresolved traumas in caregivers' own lives cause them to be more sensitive to the trauma of others, they may be more vulnerable to compassion fatigue. If caregivers have suffered cumulative losses in their lives or struggle with their feelings regarding death and dying, these are also risk factors. Note that any previous traumas or losses that caregivers have experienced are in themselves external factors, but caregivers' ongoing inner responses to them and how they have shaped who the caregivers are today are internal factors.

Perhaps caregivers have an incessant need to help others, or their self-esteem is based on "doing" rather than "being." Or maybe caregivers' personal identities are based exclusively on their professional identities. Some people are at risk because they felt isolated or disconnected from their primary caregivers as a child. Caregivers' sense of mastery and feelings of inadequacy can play a role. If caregivers have a history of mental illness, they are also at risk of developing compassion fatigue. This is not an exhaustive list but rather a sampling of some of the issues that may be at stake. The causes in any given situation will most likely be a unique mix of internal and external factors. So next, we will look at common external factors in this mix.

External Factors

External factors contributing to the development of compassion fatigue include all the factors that originate outside yourself—the circumstances in which you find yourself as you go about the practice of veterinary caregiving or even the circumstances that influenced you earlier in life. These may be external constraints, such as time, or external problems that repeatedly arise in veterinary caregiving, such as recurring loss. Past trauma may influence how caregivers react to current secondary trauma or may have shaped who they are. Work-related stresses also contribute. Again, these factors can accumulate over time. And again, they are usually mixed and intertwined. However, we'll break them down and look at each area separately.

Time Constraints

Time, or more precisely the lack thereof, is a major external contributor to compassion fatigue. Because veterinary professionals are typically overwhelmed by their schedules, their workloads, and the stresses inherent in their profession, many stop doing the very things that would help them prevent compassion fatigue. I've often seen veterinary professionals stop socializing, exploring, or participating in outside interests. Physical exercise can go by the wayside. All of this creates a vicious cycle and increases the detrimental effects of compassion fatigue.

Moreover, time is a factor because it is often the accumulation of loss and stress over time that produces compassion fatigue. Anyone can experience a bad day or a bad week, but when you have a bad year, and it is the result of compassionate caregiving without abatement through self-care strategies, you are at great risk of spiraling into compassion fatigue.

Exposure to Death and Grief

Another common contributor to compassion fatigue is continual exposure to death and grief in veterinary practice. The human-animal bond is very strong, and the sense of trauma and loss is significant when that relationship is severed. Compassionate caregivers feel that loss intensely even when they were not close to the animal that has died because they can relate deeply to the client's grief. We will look at how grief contributes to the battle with compassion fatigue in more depth in chapters 3 and 4.

Unresolved Trauma

The implication is that people who choose caregiving as their occupation sometimes learn to take on that role amid pain and suffering in their family life. Compassion fatigue can therefore stem not just from current external losses but also from external losses experienced earlier in life. This is certainly not always the case, but it is a possibility and should be considered when compassion fatigue becomes an issue.

According to Lindsay Bicknell-Hentges and John J. Lynch (2009), professors of counseling and psychology at Chicago State University, a child's age plays a significant role in the impact of stress and emotional trauma. If a traumatic event occurs during the first three years of a child's life, when brain growth is taking place in the right hemisphere, the development of "self-soothing" abilities can be disrupted. This is because communication is processed here, including nonverbal signals such as facial expressions. According to Dr. Daniel Siegel (2020), clinical professor of psychiatry at the University of California, Los Angeles, School of Medicine, childhood traumas can cause problems in adulthood related to impulse control and affect behavioral responses to strong emotions. They can lead to hypervigilance, PTSD, and other anxiety-related disorders. In my opinion, such tendencies also predispose people to compassion fatigue, particularly those who choose careers involving continual exposure to trauma and loss, such as those in veterinary care.

Work-Related Stress

Clinicians who fail to manage their work-related stress often fall victim to compassion fatigue. Work-related stresses can overwhelm the veterinary professional's ability to cope. Recall that compassion fatigue is an accumulation of stress, trauma, and loss that results from continually dealing with the pain and trauma of others. It often involves a preoccupation with the patient or client through reexperiencing the traumatic event and subsequent attempts to avoid reminders of it. Work-related stresses contribute to the overall sense of being overwhelmed and unable to cope.

Stresses in the workplace that contribute to compassion fatigue can include continual exposure to sick and dying animals as well as long hours, financial pressures, difficult interrelationships among coworkers, and poor communication in the workplace.

As with internal factors, various other external factors can apply in individual circumstances. In individual lives, there are countless triggering factors. For example, stress in an individual caregiver's personal life can play a role in compassion fatigue. Perhaps your spouse is not at all supportive of the odd hours often demanded by a veterinary practice. Cultural factors can also be at work—for instance, in some cultures or subcultures, expressing your feelings is discouraged.

It is even possible that some of those who experience compassion fatigue are not truly cut out to be veterinary caregivers; in some cases, their parents were veterinary caregivers, and there was tremendous pressure to enter the field (which is another external factor). However, this is very rare. Most external factors fit into the categories listed above in some way. Most of the time, self-care strategies can restore caregivers so that they can again enjoy their occupation.

Whatever the etiology, one thing is true: most people with compassion fatigue became veterinary care professionals because they wanted to make a difference. Most tend to put the needs of others ahead of their own. Not putting yourself first, combined with being exposed continually to the trauma of others, can lead quickly to both burnout and compassion fatigue. Suffering from the huge toll on your physical and mental health, being too busy to tend to your well-being, and putting your own needs last will undoubtedly lead you straight into an insidious battle with compassion fatigue.

For the Trainer

After reading chapter 2, either on your own or as a group, discuss the following:

1. Can you think of instances in which you noticed the phenomenon of "mirror neurons" in action when people who were interacting with each other mimicked each other's positions or attitudes? Have you noticed the phenomenon in yourself? Explain your answer to others in the group if you'd like.
2. Do you think you sometimes take on the emotions of the people around you? Share your responses on a voluntary basis.
3. Have you ever taken a personality test, such as the Myers-Briggs Type Indicator (MBTI)? Did your findings help you know yourself better? (Training suggestion: have group members complete the MBTI, then discuss results on a voluntary basis.)
4. Do you think you could benefit from assertiveness training? Why or why not? Share your answers on a voluntary basis. If you have already completed assertiveness training and feel comfortable sharing, explain to group members what it was like and what you felt you learned.

5. Try to identify internal and external factors that may put you at risk of compassion fatigue. Discuss your answers on a voluntary basis.
6. Do you think your training fully equipped you to cope with the suffering and trauma you have witnessed since becoming part of a veterinary practice team?

3

Honoring the Bond of Attachment

Grief teaches the steadiest of minds to waver.

—SOPHOCLES

The bond between a parent and child, between a husband and wife, or between any two people who are close, defines who we are. These bonds give us joy and meaning in life. They can also be a source of grief and sorrow, especially when we experience loss. The human-animal bond is similar and can be very powerful. This type of bond is also known as attachment, which John Bowlby (1969) defined as the "lasting psychological connectedness between two living things."

When veterinary caregivers witness the loss and sorrow of their clients, they feel those losses too. Because you have experienced attachments in your own life, you can relate to your clients' attachments. When clients experience fear for their animals that are ill, are distressed by their injuries, or grieve their loss, veterinary caregivers have compassion for them. They may also feel quite close to their patients and clients, and this intensifies their concern when their patients suffer. That repeated sense of trauma and intense loss is based on these attachments, and therefore, understanding attachment is an important part of the battle with compassion fatigue.

It is essential to honor the human-animal bond and to be constantly aware of it as you interact with clients. This bond is perhaps one of the two greatest contributors to compassion fatigue. (The other is euthanasia, which we look at in chapter 4.) Because of this bond, loss is felt more acutely, which leads to compassion fatigue. In this chapter, we look in more detail at the human-animal bond and examine what it means for the issue of compassion fatigue.

Pet-Owner Attachment

Often in our society, the attachments people share with their pets are the only attachment relationships they have. Children move away, leaving an "empty nest," and people are living longer lives than in the past, often alone after the death of a spouse. Young adults are often single for a longer period. Spouses divorce and find themselves single again. Children adjusting to a divorce, attending a new school, or facing peer pressures also go through periods of loneliness. In our high-tech world, despite constant contact via cell phone and social media, it has become increasingly obvious that people are lonelier than ever.

A pet may be the only relationship in which a person feels loved, appreciated, and valued. Pets often offer what human beings cannot: a sense of completely nonjudgmental and unconditional love. Because of this and the attachments we form with pets, the grieving process when a pet dies can be very much like that after the death of a human.

Your clients need support before, during, and after the loss of a pet. As a veterinary caregiver, you must take care of not only pets but also clients and families. But while doing so, you must also look after yourself. In this section, we look first at the basics of the human-animal bond and then at the grieving process. After that, we look specifically at how all of this affects the veterinary caregiver.

The Development of the Bond

Numerous studies have shown the benefits of the human-animal bond. Relationships with pets can elevate our mood, lower our blood pressure, and help our heart rate decrease. Pets can increase our self-esteem, and they can alert us to impending dangers. Contact with pets accelerates healing in humans who are ill or who have undergone surgery; it can even minimize postoperative bleeding. If this isn't enough, a variety of other benefits flow from the human-animal bond (see textbox "Therapy Animals").

The human-animal bond has been around for a long time. It goes back to ancient times, as depicted in ancient Egyptian art or cave paintings in what

Therapy Animals

Pet Partners, a program established by the Delta Society, citing numerous studies, compiled a list of many ways in which pets have been proven to aid humans in the therapeutic sense (Pet Partners 2020). Those benefiting from pet therapy included joint-replacement patients (who didn't need as much pain medication as patients who didn't receive pet therapy), patients undergoing magnetic resonance imaging scans (who were calmer than patients who didn't receive the pet therapy and required fewer sedatives), and schizophrenia patients (who felt less anxious during sessions when a therapy dog was present).

Cardiology and hypertension patients also benefited, as did people with AIDS. People living alone feel safer when they have a dog, and pet owners have fewer physical and psychological problems in general than non–pet owners. Families are generally happier after acquiring a pet. For both children and adults, interacting with dogs develops empathy and improves interaction with other humans.

The benefits go to people across the spectrum, from children to seniors. Children show substantial benefits when they have contact with pets. Pet therapy benefits children who are undergoing treatment for cancer, for example, as well as children who have experienced trauma and children with disabilities. If exposed to pets early, children have fewer allergies. Children with pets even receive better scores on tests of empathy, exhibit greater degrees of self-reliance and self-esteem, and become more nurturing.

And that's not all. Children have less stress at dentist and doctor appointments if a dog is present. They are more likely to engage in sports and other hobbies and to do their chores. They have better cognitive development. Pets even help children adjust to the illness or death of a parent.

As for seniors, the Pet Partners list cited studies showing the benefits of pets for residents of long-term care facilities, Alzheimer's patients, and hospice patients. But even healthy seniors benefit: seniors who own dogs go to the doctor less often, have more active lifestyles, and have lower levels of stress in daily life.

With all this evidence to support the benefits of the human-animal bond, it is no wonder that when pets are sick or injured or when pets die, their owners undergo a grieving process. As a veterinary caregiver, your compassion for them is also strong, and over time, this compassion fatigue can overwhelm you.

is now France. In some ways, animals and humans have evolved together. Dogs have been bred to do a variety of tasks for humans, including shepherding and hunting, and have therefore interacted with humans in everyday life for centuries.

For all these reasons, the human-animal bond is very strong. Many pet owners feel that their pets are like members of the family. This affects how they feel when their pets are ill or injured and how they grieve for them when they die. The stronger the bond and the more intense the relationship, the greater the fear of losing the animal and the grief when that relationship must end.

The Bond and the Grieving Process

The grief that results from the loss of a pet can often equal or even exceed the grief that results from the loss of a human relationship. Pet owners can find themselves feeling confused and even guilty when they experience a more devastating and difficult recovery from the loss of a pet than they did from the death of a close family member. But the reasons for this are not so difficult to understand. Where else do we find a relationship where we can be fully authentic at all times and not be judged for it? How many people accept us for who we are, no matter how we look, what sort of mood we're in, or how much money we make? Often, it is our four-legged family members that fill this role.

Through all of this, the attachment between the pet owner and the pet grows, especially if the pet owner doesn't have a strong social support system. It doesn't matter how or why a pet dies, whether the pet lived a long life or a short life, whether the pet passed suddenly or the decision to euthanize was made. The pain that results is a natural consequence of the intensity of losing a relationship with one's source of nonjudgmental companionship and unconditional love.

Your clients who are grieving the loss of a pet need your compassion. They need someone who cares and is willing to listen. You should know how to help them through it (see textbox "Helping Clients Who Are Grieving" in chapter 4). But remember that you, too, are affected. As you invest your emotional resources into your grieving clients, you may become vulnerable to compassion fatigue, unless you know how to shield yourself from it (see textbox "Case Study: Dr. Bell"). I highly suggest taking the human-animal bond training offered by the American Animal Hospital Association (AAHA) and Human Animal Bond Academy (HABA).

Case Study | Dr. Bell

Dr. Bell, a highly respected specialist in veterinary medicine, is a warm and compassionate doctor, and his clients and staff rely on his expertise as well as on his kind and gentle nature. Lately, however, his practice has seen an unusual number of very traumatic cases. Consequently, Dr. Bell has been experiencing the emotional distress of three different families. He is very fond of all of them. To make matters worse, his own dog, a cherished twelve-year-old border collie, recently lost a battle with her own disease.

Being the good doctor that he is—and the one everyone can lean on—Dr. Bell forced himself to go to work the day after losing his beloved pet, and he continued to stick to his routine. His wife begged him to take some time off, and he refused. But she began to see some warning signs, and her husband began to seem like a completely different person. At work, he tried desperately to act as if nothing were wrong and continued to be available to meet everyone else's needs. But at home, he became sullen, angry, and withdrawn. He isolated himself from friends and family, preferring to stay in bed or, at most, to plop himself in front of the TV. Eventually, Dr. Bell tried to end his own life. Fortunately, he survived, and the suicide attempt became a wake-up call for him to get help.

Sadly, however, this isn't an uncommon scenario. When a veterinary caregiver who is already battling the symptoms of compassion fatigue is suddenly confronted by personal losses, the factors can pile up to produce a very dangerous situation. Many of us don't seem to be able to give ourselves the same compassion that we give so readily to others.

Forcing ourselves to have to be okay when we are not only serves to increase our stress, anxiety, and symptoms of depression. If you get nothing else from this book, please get this: you must take care of yourself on an ongoing and consistent basis if you want to continue in a career surrounded by trauma. If you do not take care of yourself, you are not going to be able to take care of anyone else, including your patients, clients, family, and friends. You are no different from anyone else in that you need and deserve the support of others when grieving your own losses.

Attachment and Grief in Veterinary Caregiving

When a client's pet dies, you, too, are affected by the loss. You have bonded to some extent with the animal yourself, and you are also taking on some of the client's pain. Furthermore, you are called on to do this repeatedly. Over time, if compassion fatigue is not prevented, it must be addressed.

As a team member of a veterinary practice, you probably remember how significant various animals have been in your own life. You have firsthand experience of the human-animal bond because you have been on the human side of that bond. Perhaps you had a pet as a child that was very important to you. That pet may have been a close companion. If you were a 4-H club member or participated in equestrian activities, the animals in your life may have been paramount.

Because you had these experiences, you know how your clients feel when their beloved animals are ill or injured, or when they have died or must be euthanized. This is what enables you to have compassion. These deep feelings go right to the heart of what drew you into the veterinary field. Perhaps as a youth you saw an animal die, and you wanted to stop that from happening; you wanted to heal the animal and keep other people from experiencing the same kind of grief that you experienced.

But in veterinary practice—as in any medical field—healing is not always possible. And when you see pets dying and clients grieving, you may feel inadequate. You may question whether you could have done something differently or, if you tend to be a perfectionist, berate yourself for not saving the pet's life. Compassion fatigue results when your deeply felt sense of compassion for others—often earned through your own grief that was intimately connected to a human-animal bond—brings you to the breaking point. The constant exposure to the suffering of others becomes exhausting. You seem to never get relief from it, and it begins to affect you so much that you experience the symptoms described in chapter 1, such as anger, irritability, apathy, and sleep disturbances. It is so exhausting, in part because it makes you question your self-worth and identity and causes you to recall times when you yourself were grieving.

Later in this book, I will show you how to take care of yourself to prevent this process from progressing to compassion fatigue. But next, we look at the second major cause of compassion fatigue: euthanasia.

The human-animal bond is a wonderful thing. In our relationships with animals, we celebrate life and connection. But when you experience repeated loss and are so intimately connected to the loss of others, it seems as if that vibrancy is replaced by sadness. When you witness the loss of the human-animal bond repeatedly, compassion fatigue is the natural result—unless you learn to prevent it through specific strategies discussed later in this book.

For the Trainer

After reading chapter 3, either on your own or as a group, discuss the following:

1. Recall an animal with which you had a strong bond, perhaps as a child. How would you describe this bond?
2. Did this bond play a role in your decision to enter veterinary practice? Do your memories of this pet help you relate to your clients?
3. Did you experience the loss of that pet? Do you recall how you felt when that loss occurred?
4. If you did experience the loss of a beloved pet, would you say the attachment was still worth it despite the loss? Recall the good times you had with that pet as well. Describe to group members one of your best memories of that pet.

4

Euthanasia and Its Emotional Impact on the Team

Dream as if you'll live forever, live as if you'll die today.

—JAMES DEAN

Euthanasia is emotionally taxing for clients and veterinary team members alike. If veterinarians and team members can understand what clients are experiencing and guide them through this challenging time, clients will come through the experience more positively, and all involved will likely be less prone to compassion fatigue. It is possible to handle euthanasia in an authentic way, respect the human-animal bond, and allow for emotions and grief to be expressed.

The client receives strength and comfort from this approach, leaving veterinary caregivers feeling that they did help the client after all. The pet may have died, but the importance of the pet's life and the client's relationship with the pet were honored. This kind of ending for the pet's life is not only good for the client but can also reduce the risk of developing compassion fatigue.

Pet Owners and Euthanasia

Euthanasia of a pet is one of life's most painful yet loving and unselfish acts. And yet the decision not to allow a cherished pet to suffer is always inherently painful. Most often, by the time your clients have decided to euthanize, they have done everything they could to save their pet's life or quality of life.

They are now at a point where the only gift they can offer is letting the pet go. Euthanasia is a promise of no more pain.

Nothing we can say will take away the pain our clients are feeling at the enormity of their loss at the time of euthanasia. However, we can take some steps to minimize the pain for the animal and the client. When we approach euthanasia this way, the client will do better, and you will feel you have helped.

For example, ensure that clients with euthanasia appointments for their pets do not wait in the same waiting room as clients with healthy pets. Instead, you can immediately escort these clients and pets into the treatment room. Have a separate entrance and waiting room, if possible, or instruct clients to call from their cell phone when arriving in the clinic's parking lot so that you can come out to help them in. Whichever method you choose, ensure these clients and pets enter a room immediately after entering your facility.

If possible, designate one room of the hospital to be a "comfort room." These rooms should contain drinking water; plenty of Kleenex; scissors and plastic baggies in case the client would like to keep a clipping of hair or fur; a warm, fuzzy blanket; a large pet bed or a pillow large enough for clients to sit or lie on with their pets; a CD player to play soft music during or after the procedure; and a dimmer switch, if possible, to keep the lighting soft. Because the sound of water is calming, you might also consider having a small fountain in the room as part of the decor.

This is potentially one of the most difficult decisions your client has ever had to make, and it must be met with compassion and kindness by everyone on the veterinary care team. Escorting clients immediately into a room and having a blanket for the pet to lie on speaks volumes to the client. Staff members entering the room should take a deep breath first and slow down a bit. It is important to be respectful and sensitive. The goal at this time is to be caring and personal and to make a connection with the client, not to be efficient. If the client does not already know team members who enter the room, team members should be sure to introduce themselves. Choose your words carefully and ensure they will not make clients feel even worse than they already do.

Most clients wish to be present for the euthanasia, but confirm this before the appointment. If a client would rather not be present, honor this decision. If the client is present, take the time to explain everything you are doing before and during the euthanasia procedure. For example, inform the client beforehand that the pet's eyes won't close, that the pet might take one long last breath, and that it is common for pets to urinate or defecate while passing. After sedating the pet, give your client some time, and then ask the client if they are ready for you to give the pet the final injection. Don't be afraid to use touch; it is a powerful tool in healing. After the final injection and after you have checked the pet's heart, put a hand on the client's hand or shoulder and say gently, "she's gone" or "he's passed."

Compassion and caring can make all the difference in the world when we are in the midst of losing a loved one. Give your clients as much time as they need to say goodbye to their pets after euthanasia, and avoid trying to rush them. If the client has brought music to play, allow the music to stay on as long as the client would like.

The worst thing we can do when people are grieving is to minimize their feelings, tell them what to do or how to feel, advise getting another pet, or throw well-known but inappropriate clichés at them such as "don't worry, time heals all," "God doesn't give us more than we can handle," "he's better off where he is," or "you should be grateful, he was really old, and he had a good life." I call that pouring salt into the wound. "Of course he had a good and long life," most of us would think. "But that only makes it harder, not easier, because we spent all those wonderful years together, and my life revolved around him, and now he's gone."

Your clients will probably run across some of these salt pourers among their friends and relatives. Although their words can hurt, I don't believe that the pourers of salt are malicious. Often they haven't had the privilege and joy of sharing a bond with a four-legged family member, and their ignorance propels them to say such things. I choose to feel sorry for such people rather than angry, and I suggest that those who are grieving do the same.

Ours is a difficult society in which to grieve, and it is perhaps one of the loneliest societies in the world. When I volunteered in the orphanage in India operated by Mother Teresa, she once said to me, "No more adoptions to the United States. You can continue to send to Denmark, Norway, Sweden, and Italy, but no more adoptions to the U.S." I had several wonderful American families waiting for babies, and I was puzzled and concerned. I asked her why she was making this decision. She replied, "Because of the poverty." "Mother," I said, "we are standing in the middle of Calcutta, and you are talking about the poverty of my country?" "No, no, no," she said, shaking her finger back and forth. "You have it wrong." She then pointed to her heart, saying, "The poverty is here. I have never been in a more lonely country than the United States, and I don't want my babies being raised there."

Sadly, I knew that Mother Teresa was correct. The United States can be a very lonely society. People find comfort in their pets, but pet loss is often unrecognized and unacknowledged. Because a pet, for many people, is their

Helping Clients Who Are Grieving

Are you feeling powerless? Let me assure you, you are not. By simply being there and listening to your grieving clients with an empathetic ear, you are offering them an avenue to begin the healing process.

The grieving process is different for everyone; your clients are the only ones who know how they feel. Don't make the mistake of trying to tell someone how to feel. The best way to support people who are grieving is to listen and help them normalize their feelings. People feel what they feel. These feelings must be honored, heard, and validated. Please resist the temptation to judge clients or compare them to others.

Helping veterinary clients who have experienced loss can be very challenging. Because the grieving process is unique to every individual, there is no one protocol to follow. These clients may experience a wide range of emotions. They can be hypervigilant, appreciative, apprehensive, hypersensitive, or emotional. They may act protective and defensive or feel vulnerable and frightened. They may become angry, controlling, manipulative, and even suicidal when their sense of safety is threatened. It's important to understand that these negative reactions are survival mechanisms that surface when one feels out of control or unsafe. When such behaviors are projected toward you, remember not to personalize them.

You might begin to feel frustrated with clients who do not seem to get better, who call you continually or say the same things repeatedly. Although feeling this way is normal and understandable, try not to allow your frustration to show. Let clients know you can see how hard this is for them, and then refer them to a specialist. It may be time to call in an expert in grief recovery. With the client's permission, give the specialist the client's phone number so the specialist can follow up.

---

only source of love, companionship, and affection, losing a pet can be catastrophic, leading to all sorts of pathological responses. When a human dies, those who mourn can receive support and understanding through family gatherings, words of sympathy, and religious rituals. But when a pet dies, these things are missing, leaving the grieving pet owner without support.

As veterinary caregivers, we must attempt to fill this gap. To lend comfort and support to grieving people, one of the best things we can do is listen. Develop your listening skills so that you can provide these for your clients (see

Listen Up

How to Help Grieving Clients by Listening

It is essential for veterinary caregivers to know how to be good listeners. Listening is one of the most effective ways to express compassion and help clients work through their grief. Follow these suggestions when listening to clients who have lost a pet:

- Be **completely engaged** by being fully present when listening to someone describing their pain or trauma. Grievers are typically hypervigilant and will therefore notice if the listener is no longer paying full attention. Listening without having to fix the problem, without interrupting, and without feeling the need to impose our own stories (unless they would benefit the bereaved) is an important skill.
- We can also convey a sense of concern and care by using **active and/or reflective listening skills** to let grievers know we are truly hearing them. To do this, we repeat to clients some of the most important points they conveyed. For example, you might say, "So, let me see if I got this straight. The part you are struggling with the most right now is the last memory that you had when your loved one was taken from you and put into the intensive care unit at the emergency clinic. Is that right?" This technique allows the grieving client to correct any miscommunications or misunderstandings. It also conveys that you are interested and listening.
- **Reflective listening** goes even deeper, conveying to clients that the listener values and understands them. With this technique, you reflect back on what clients say and the feelings you believe they are experiencing. In reflective listening, you might say, for example, "So, let me see if I got this straight. You are not only struggling with the last image you had of your loved one going into the intensive care unit at the emergency clinic, but you are also feeling very guilty and angry at yourself for not having taken her the day before to her regular veterinarian when you had the first inkling that something wasn't right. Is that correct?" When we use reflective listening, our clients feel valued and important because we took the time to truly understand.
- Be aware of **body language**, yours and the client's. Body language conveys a lot of information. Uncross your arms and face the client. If you are sitting, try to be on the client's level. Maintain eye contact. If the client cries, do not jump up immediately and grab the Kleenex because this could

convey your discomfort with their tears; instead, continue listening, and if the client appears to be searching for a tissue, gently and slowly get up and place it next to them, then quietly and unassumingly go back to where you were sitting.

- Many psychologists and bereavement counselors believe not showing your tears in the room is important, but I can't entirely agree. I believe that if you are overcome with emotion, it's fine to let it show. Your nonverbal message of emotion will speak to how much you care about the client and the pet, which can be a great source of comfort to the client. That does not mean you should wail uncontrollably; it simply means that if tears well up naturally, you should not try to stop them.

textboxes "Helping Clients Who Are Grieving" and "Listen Up: How to Help Grieving Clients by Listening").

Many people who have grieved the loss of a pet have told me over the years that they would remain ever faithful to the veterinary practice that provided them with grief support. Many credited the practice with helping them find their way back after the death of a beloved pet. These communication skills are very valuable. Keep in mind that they require you to be completely open and available to your client's stories. Also, keep in mind that these stories do place you in harm's way by subjecting you to the client's trauma and, thereby, compassion fatigue. It is normal to experience a wide range of emotions surrounding euthanasia, and we will discuss these in the next section.

Be creative in how you handle euthanasia. For example, many practices offer to make paw prints for clients whose pets are undergoing euthanasia. Consider suggesting your client bring pictures of the pet to the practice to post on a bulletin board or add to a photo album. Take a few minutes to allow the client to show you some of these pictures. Some clients may wish to read a poem before or after the procedure or decide to commemorate the pet's life later on in some other way.

If children are involved, they might like to draw a picture of the pet during a happy time or draw a picture or write a letter to send with the pet. Have a few children's books on pet loss available in case children are present. Answer children's questions honestly while remembering that the fewer words, the better for younger children. Children are typically not seeking lengthy explanations; often, a simple yes or no is all they need to feel comforted.

Send a sympathy card that all team members sign to arrive a few days later, and make a follow-up call to see how the client is doing. Before the day of the euthanasia appointment, let clients know their options for handling the pet's body, ask what their preference is, and offer to arrange for any details that may be necessary for cremation or burial. Be sure that the pet's body is treated with dignity and respect at all times.

Euthanasia and Veterinary Professionals

Although you are a professional, you must also permit yourself to grieve when a patient dies. It is normal for a veterinary caregiver to go through a wide range of emotions, from confusion and sadness to fatigue and sometimes even a sense of relief, typically accompanied by a significant amount of guilt. Because you are responsible for caring for the needs of pets, you cannot help but form strong attachments to some of them, which predisposes you to your own experiences of grief and loss as well as compassion fatigue.

Although emotions are normal, that does not make having these feelings fun, pleasant, or easy. Feelings of frustration and powerlessness may come up for you, especially if you had to be involved in ending a life that you spent a lot of time and energy trying to save. You may feel as though you have no sense of control because the animal died anyway even after all the time and energy you invested in that particular pet. You may feel emotional pain if the pet didn't die as you would have wanted. You may feel anger or tension with other members of the practice team or a veterinarian at a different hospital who played a role in the pet's care. You may feel as if no one is handling the situation correctly or struggle with boundary issues over how much time you should spend with your clients.

Most of all, you are likely to be emotionally overwhelmed by how frequently you are forced to deal with trauma and the loss of your patients. Finding, facing, and healing any personal issues that may be compelling you to take on more than you should can ultimately be what saves you.

Whether veterinary professionals have been trained or prepared to work in trauma and loss is not what determines their experiences while working with such emotionally difficult situations. As mentioned earlier, most veterinary professionals enter the field because of their love for animals. So, expecting continual exposure to euthanasia not to have a profoundly negative effect on every level of the veterinary profession is naïve at best. Support staff are often on the front line with clients as they go through the before-and-after impact of their traumatic loss. Managing such negative emotions without damaging yourself or your relationships is the goal.

Even when euthanasia goes well, the emotional impact can have an enormous effect on you. Even if you have participated in many euthanasia procedures, no two go precisely the same way, and there is no guarantee they will go the way you want them to. When the unexpected occurs, maintain a calm attitude and make the best decision possible (see textbox "Case Study: Julia").

There is a high degree of emotional trauma, career burnout, and compassion fatigue among veterinarians who must perform euthanasia frequently. One of the most stressful situations reported by veterinarians across the board involves requests for euthanasia on perfectly healthy pets or pets that could benefit from veterinary care, but the owners opt for euthanasia anyway. Sometimes they do not have the funds to pay for treatment; sometimes they do not believe in doing complicated medical procedures on pets. More tragic situations such as this are seen during economic downturns than when the

Case Study | Julia

I was once called on to assist with the euthanasia of a sixteen-year-old poodle named Julia, who had been physically shutting down for weeks. Blind and deaf for years, this little trooper had developed heart and kidney problems, and then a large tumor was discovered near her liver. Her decline was rapid. She stopped eating (previously her favorite pastime), slept most of the time, and was weak and shaky. By the time I arrived to pick her up for her final moments with her person, she hadn't eaten for two weeks and couldn't stand up without falling over.

I wrapped her in a blanket and took her to the appointment on the lap of her loved one. It wasn't easy to ascertain whether she was still alive; I thought she might have already passed by the time we reached the veterinarian's office. However, when the veterinarian administered the first syringe of euthanasia drugs, our little three-pound poodle simply kept breathing. I felt horrible for the veterinarian—this unexpected turn of events visibly shook her. The client was even more distressed and confused. Eventually, this incredible and caring professional, who has helped literally hundreds of pets pass peacefully, returned to the room with yet another syringe, and the breathing was no more.

The moral of the story is this: expect the unexpected. Don't let it rattle you; do your best with the circumstances given to you.

economy is strong. As a veterinary caregiver, you may find it extremely difficult to euthanize pets you know did not have to die.

Also stressful and frustrating are situations in which a client is not prepared to let go of a pet that is obviously suffering and no longer enjoys what you believe is an acceptable quality of life. In these cases, pet-loss professionals can sometimes help. They can be called in as an additional voice of reason to counsel the client, but this process can also be very emotionally taxing.

Clients sometimes have a hard time knowing when to let go. Blinded by their love for their pet or their fear of loss, many cannot recognize the suffering before them. Grief can be physical, mental, or emotional, or it can involve the loss of one's dignity. A pet-loss professional can help the client recognize this (see textbox "Case Study: Don").

The AVMA, in its "Guidelines for the Euthanasia of Animals" (2020a), referred to needing to consider human psychological responses to euthanasia when helping clients make this decision and when administering euthanasia. The guidelines state that grief is the most common reaction. The AVMA also recognizes that veterinary team members "become attached to patients and struggle with the ethics of the caring-killing paradox, particularly when they must end the lives of animals they have known and treated for many years."

Moreover, a quantitative investigation, "The Caring-Killing Paradox," performed by a team at the University of North Carolina at Charlotte (Reeve et al. 2005), revealed the psychological ramifications of euthanasia-related employment. They found that euthanasia-related stress is prevalent and associated with increased substance use, somatic complaints, overall job stress, conflicts in relationships (including family and personal), and lower levels of job satisfaction. According to the authors, "Analyses provided evidence that euthanasia-related work has a significant negative relation with employee wellbeing independent of its relation with generalized job stress. Exploratory analyses also suggest that individual, work, and organizational differences may influence perceived stress and appear to be associated with certain aspects of employee wellbeing."

How we work, how we perceive our work, our temperaments, and the level of emotional support we receive in our employment settings all influence how well we handle continual exposure to death and trauma through euthanasia as veterinary team members. Euthanasia can potentially affect all veterinary team members, causing enormous emotional difficulty. These painful and traumatic experiences begin at the reception desk and affect every team member. Here are some of the implications.

Case Study | Don

A few years ago, I received a call from Don, who asked whether I would make a house call. He wanted to pay me to come out and assess his cat to help him determine whether it was time to euthanize. I explained that I was not a veterinarian and did not have the skills to make such a determination, to which he quickly replied that he was aware of that but had heard that I had assisted with in-home euthanasia. He thought that I was the right person to ask. He wanted my opinion from a strictly spiritual standpoint.

Don said that he had previously consulted three veterinarians who concurred that the cat would make no improvement and that any time would be short. I agreed to meet with him, and when I got to his house, the man greeted me at the door and promptly introduced me to his beloved pet.

The cat, unable to move, was lying on her right side and barely noticed a stranger bent over her, speaking her name. "Watch this," said Don. "She still loves it when I take her outside." With giant, loving hands, he gently scooped her up into his arms, where she lay motionless on their journey. I followed him back out the front door to a patch of grass with a tree that divided his house from the next.

Don laid his precious one down on the soft grass. "There, you see?" he said. "Can you see how her eyes lit up? She still loves being outdoors. You can see it, can't you?" he begged. Sadly, I couldn't see it. I saw the mere shell of a former proud and beautiful cat with no dignity left. What I saw was sadness or, worse, emptiness. If I were to guess, the only thing that kept that beautiful cat from passing was her concern for the welfare of her person.

I had to tell Don what I saw, and it broke my heart to speak the words he feared so much. To his credit, he listened. He understood what I was saying, and when he combined that with the medical information from the three veterinarians, he was able to make the necessary call. An appointment was set for that evening to help his cat make her final transition. The in-home euthanasia veterinarian arrived four hours later, and I finally left his home three hours after that.

It was excruciatingly painful for this man to lose his cat because he had no one left on this earth to whom he felt close. The veterinarian called me the next morning and asked for time to debrief. She said she wasn't sure why, but this case had really gotten to her. She had found herself unable to sleep all night.

Front-Office Staff

These invaluable team members are typically not trained in death and dying or euthanasia, yet they define our practices by how they interact with every client who walks through the front door. Seldom do practices take the time to train front-office personnel thoroughly in this regard, nor do they acknowledge their loss when a valued or favorite patient dies. However, they, too, form relationships with the patients and clients and can suffer from compassion fatigue. They should be included in training surrounding euthanasia and compassion fatigue issues (see textbox "Case Study: Chris").

Case Study | Chris

Chris, a receptionist, was a tremendous asset to the practice where she worked. Kind, professional, highly competent, and compassionate, she decided she could not continue in her career much longer. She had found that caring too much in the veterinary field could be a detriment rather than an asset.

Because she cared so much, Chris had gotten to the point where she felt she couldn't deal with another traumatic loss or uncaring owner. She could not watch one more pet with whom she had formed a relationship being escorted down the hallway, knowing that the animal would never return because its family had given up on the pet. She admitted to trying to intercede on more than one occasion to advocate for a pet that she felt was getting the short end of the stick.

Chris's final straw was a sweet Newfoundland who was "an outside dog," never having lived inside a home. The dog, quite obviously, was never groomed or bathed. Chris said that the dog had foxtails and mats by the dozens and was absolutely filthy. The owner, claiming to have allergies, never touched the dog without wearing plastic gloves. This poor, sweet dog never knew the comforts of a home or of being touched affectionately.

Chris could barely contain herself and offered to have the dog groomed at no cost to the client. She had spoken to the staff and found two other individuals, an assistant and an off-duty technician, who offered their work for free. The client, who was retired and lived alone, said she did not want to take the time to wait.

That was it for Chris, the final straw. The veterinary profession thereby lost a true asset. Chris said that her caring impeded her from being able to stay in the industry she had thought she would love. She had come to the painful realization that she needed to separate her occupation from her passion, animal care and advocacy.

Technicians

Technicians typically have a vast number of responsibilities. They often find themselves in highly stressful situations. They are forced to multitask most of the time, and they also have to communicate with clients on highly sensitive issues, including euthanasia.

Even though technicians are typically comfortable with the idea that euthanasia can help alleviate suffering, some euthanasia procedures are far more traumatic than others. Some technicians with several years of experience have reported feeling uncomfortable about the number of euthanasia procedures in which they have participated. Others have reported struggling with ethical dilemmas when they assisted veterinarians with whom they had not previously worked. In these cases, they found they had a completely different philosophy from the veterinarians about euthanasia options.

Some technicians leave practices for this reason, and I know one who left the field altogether. In my experience, many technicians find two types of euthanasia procedures especially difficult emotionally. These are intracardiac euthanasia, in which a needle is injected directly into the pet's heart, and the "old-school" procedure, as it is commonly called, whereby the euthanasia solution is injected without the benefit of a previously administered sedative or anesthesia to allow the pet to relax or fall asleep first.

Interns

The typical veterinary intern also has a considerable number of responsibilities and must communicate with emotional clients on sensitive issues such as euthanasia. Interns typically have no time for themselves and are often sleep deprived. The idea of self-care is but a distant dream. Because they are often physically and emotionally exhausted, these caring individuals can become overemotional when dealing with a difficult euthanasia. If you are an intern, it is essential for you to realize this. Prepare yourself properly before entering the room, and practice tiny increments of proactive self-care whenever and wherever possible.

Groomers

Groomers can have very intense relationships with the pets they care for on a consistent basis. They may see them monthly for many years. They may even be the ones to discover a small lump and hence a dog's cancer because they are the ones lathering dogs up and massaging shampoo into their fur. In these cases, they may also be the ones to relay the frightening information to pet owners. The whirlwind of diagnosis, treatment plans, and protocols then begins, and the groomer receives updates about the dog's health as grooming continues, possibly becoming the pet owner's primary confidant. As a result, groomers can be consumed by grief. Their compassion for the dog and owner can lead to compassion fatigue.

Behaviorists

Behaviorists must form close relationships with the pets with which they work. They often know the pets better than anyone else and find themselves acting as a voice for the pet, creating an even closer bond between them. When a pet with which behaviorists have been working dies, the behaviorists typically experience grief and may feel guilty. The guilt stems from the misconception that they "somehow should have known."

"Should haves" and "shouldn't haves" are common in grief and loss; I have rarely met a bereaved individual who did not have them (see textbox "Should

Should Haves and Shouldn't Haves

Behaviorists, as well as pet owners, are prone to question themselves about what they should or shouldn't have done for a pet that has died. Avoid this kind of self-questioning. If you find yourself saying such things, remind yourself that you did the best you could with what you knew at the time, likewise if you hear a client saying these things. We can all see more in retrospect than we can during a situation, and it is not fair to yourself to judge your behavior with the knowledge of hindsight.

Here are some typical "should haves" and "shouldn't haves": "I shouldn't have taken him to the dog park"; "I should have spent more time with her"; "I should have taken her to the doctor sooner"; "I shouldn't have left her at the emergency clinic"; "I should have gone to a specialist"; "I should never have gone to that specialist"; "I shouldn't have let them do that surgery"; "I should have let them do the surgery"; "I shouldn't have allowed the gardener to put the fertilizer on the lawn"; "I should never have allowed her in the backyard alone"; "I should have taken him on more walks"; "I should have realized sooner that something was wrong"; "I should never have gone on that vacation"; "I should never have moved." You get the idea: I could write a book on just the "should haves" and "shouldn't haves" that can be associated with grief, loss, and trauma.

Haves and Shouldn't Haves"). Even though they are common, they only make people feel worse. It is one more way to beat themselves up emotionally, which only makes their recovery even more difficult.

Euthanasia, Attitudes About Death, and Suicide

The frequency of euthanasia in veterinary care contributes to compassion fatigue, as we have seen, and if this compassion fatigue continues without abatement, it can progress to something worse. Ultimately, it can in some cases lead to suicide. Is there a more specific connection here? Does euthanasia somehow affect caregivers' attitudes toward death, making suicide seem more viable when they experience intense suffering?

As one article on this issue pointed out, euthanasia must be "explained, encouraged, and justified to clients" so often that veterinary caregivers may well find that their attitudes toward death do change (Schultz 2008). This may cause caregivers to lower their inhibitions toward suicide and see it as a viable solution for dealing with their own problems.

Another article, which spurred my interest and concern about veterinary compassion fatigue in 2008, reported that the suicide rate among veterinarians in the United Kingdom was proportionally four times that of the general population and twice that of other health professionals (Bartram and Baldwin 2008). According to the authors, "Job stresses, lethal drug access, and euthanasia acceptance are among the potential driving forces behind DVMs' heightened risk."

A study by the Centers for Disease Control and Prevention (CDC), published in the *Journal of the American Veterinary Medical Association*, revealed that veterinarians in the United States are at increased risk of suicide. Female veterinarians were found to be 3.5 times more likely to commit suicide than the general population, while their male colleagues were 2.1 times more likely to take their own lives (Tomasi et al. 2019). One of the reasons for the high number of veterinary suicides I previously cited is the proximity to euthanasia drugs. That has not changed since the first edition of this book was published. Neither has the fact that veterinary professionals are at the mercy of clients who viciously attack and seek to destroy them on social media. The study also listed anxieties such as high student loan balances, long hours combined with poor pay, and the lack of balance between private lives and work as reasons for the continued high suicide rates (Tomasi et al. 2019).

Because lethal medication is so readily available in veterinary medicine, when veterinary caregivers commit suicide, it is often through deliberate drug ingestion. Veterinary caregivers not only have access to these drugs but know how to use them to end life. Intentional overdoses accounted for approximately 82 percent of veterinary suicides in the United Kingdom and only 33 percent of suicides in the general population (Bartram and Baldwin 2008).

The connection these researchers made between euthanasia and suicide is alarming, and it highlights the importance of compassion fatigue prevention and recovery techniques.

Next, our focus will shift to identifying the symptoms, paving the way for addressing and treating compassion fatigue.

For the Trainer

Discuss the following after reading chapter 4 on your own or as a group. This time, we include both discussion and an active listening exercise:

1. Share ideas about how to help clients during a euthanasia procedure. Have you tried something that seemed to work well? If so, share it with the group.
2. Try forming pairs and doing a listening exercise. For example, have a member of each pair tell the other member a story and see how many details the listener can remember. Then switch roles. As the listener, remember to be wholly engaged, to use active or reflective listening techniques, and to reflect on the speaker's feelings. Report back to the group after the exercise. Which techniques worked best for you?
3. Have you ever found yourself in a difficult situation that involved a euthanasia decision? For example, perhaps the client did not make the same decision you would have if the pet had been yours. How did you handle that conflict?
4. Are there suggestions in this chapter about how to approach euthanasia that you think would help prevent compassion fatigue from developing in veterinary caregivers?
5. What would you do if you felt a colleague was considering suicide?

5

Recognizing the Symptoms of Compassion Fatigue

Character cannot be developed in ease and quiet. Only through experiences of trial and suffering can the soul be strengthened, vision cleared, ambition inspired, and success achieved.

—HELEN KELLER

In any of the animal-care professions, caregivers need to care for themselves. This must be done proactively—not by waiting for the symptoms to appear. Learn about compassion fatigue before you ever start to have it, or you may have to learn about it the hard way. You owe it to yourself to make sure you know how to recognize what compassion fatigue looks like when it first begins, how to cope with it, and how to prevent it by finding a safe place to process and release emotions on a continual basis.

Like so many painful experiences in life, compassion fatigue is a completely individualized experience. No two people experience it in the same way. For this reason, you must learn to be aware of what your body is telling you, for that is the first place you will notice compassion fatigue manifesting itself.

The Symptoms of Compassion Fatigue

Sadly, most caregivers do not take the time to shield themselves from the potential consequences of compassion fatigue because denial is one of its primary symptoms. If you are wondering whether you have compassion fatigue, look at your recent behaviors and ask yourself the following questions. If you answer yes to the majority of the questions, you are most likely already in the clutches of compassion fatigue.

- Do you often wake up after a full night's sleep still feeling exhausted, no matter how much sleep you get?
- Does your work often feel endless and thankless?
- Do you often struggle with gut-wrenching grief?
- Has your job performance gone down?
- Do you ever feel numb or empty?
- Have you seen more problems arising in your personal relationships? Do you struggle more often with your professional relationships?
- Do you no longer have time for the activities you once enjoyed?
- Do you forget to take time to nurture yourself?
- Do you take more sick days now than when you first started in the profession?
- Do you feel guilty a lot?
- Are you feeling overwhelmed?
- Are you angrier or more easily irritated than you used to be?
- Do you find yourself turning more and more to substances to help numb you or to help you cope?
- Are you plagued with nightmares?
- Do you have trouble getting to sleep or staying asleep?
- Have you seen significant changes in your appetite?
- Do you make unhealthy food choices as a means of comfort more often than you used to?
- Do you find yourself canceling on your friends and withdrawing more and more from social contact?
- Do you often feel unsafe?
- Do you find yourself becoming impatient more often than usual?

With the massive emotional and physical demands of the veterinary profession, coupled with the self-imposed pressure of your high standards—and adding in the financial pressures that affect clients and their treatment decisions—it's no wonder that compassion fatigue is so common in veterinary care today. There seems to be a perception, particularly among caregivers, that there is not enough time to do all that must be done, especially regarding taking care of ourselves. We seem to be able to justify eliminating the things that benefit us, including having alone time, exercising, spending time with friends or family, meditating, or making time just to be and not have to do anything at all. In the long run, however, we are doing ourselves and our loved ones no favors by letting these things go by the wayside. Compassion fatigue causes high turnover rates, increases the likelihood of stress-related illnesses, results in more sick days, and in general decreases our overall productivity.

Your work as a veterinary care provider is emotionally complex and can be exhausting. Many of you struggle daily to function in environments filled with gut-wrenching trauma. Although it was once rewarding, your work can now seem both endless and thankless. You might encounter intermittent or continual feelings of guilt, deep sorrow, anger, and rage. Working with traumatized people and animals often makes care providers question their sense of safety, predictability, control, and protection. Compassion fatigue can mimic the symptoms of PTSD, including avoidance of trauma reminders or triggers, emotional numbness, nightmares, social withdrawal, and emotional flooding.

In emotional flooding, repressed fears and feelings can surface suddenly, resulting in overwhelming emotions, especially negative ones. This can lead to various detrimental behaviors, such as missing work and feeling that one's emotions are entirely out of control. For instance, in an emotional-flooding experience, one veterinary professional crawled inside one of the intensive care cages and refused to come out; she alternated between laughing hysterically and crying uncontrollably. A bright and dedicated individual, this outstanding team member had fallen victim to compassion fatigue.

You owe it to yourself to learn how to cope with the difficult emotions that are part and parcel of veterinary caregiving and find a safe place to process and release these emotions. If you do not, you may distance yourself physically and emotionally from the work you previously enjoyed and felt you were meant to do.

Get in touch with where you hold pain and stress in your body. For some, it's a stiffening and soreness of the neck; for others, it's a pain in the stomach or lower back; and for still others, it can be a tightening of the jaw. Again, everyone is different. The important thing is that you begin to notice how your body responds to stress and stores painful emotions.

Symptoms of compassion fatigue vary but commonly include the following:

- Uncharacteristic anger and/or anxiety
- Physical and/or mental exhaustion
- Chronic physical ailments
- Bottled-up emotions
- The increased impulse to rescue a pet or a person
- Paranoia
- Sadness
- Apathy
- Lowered self-esteem
- Excessive complaints about coworkers
- Receiving excessive complaints from coworkers
- Sleep and/or appetite disturbances
- No longer being able to balance objectivity with empathy
- Difficulty concentrating and staying on task
- Nightmares or flashbacks, in some cases recurring ones
- Becoming accident prone
- Substance abuse
- Excessive blaming
- Persistent headaches, neck aches, and/or stomach complaints
- Uncharacteristic tardiness
- Poor hygiene or self-care
- A sense of vulnerability, sadness, apathy, or impending doom
- An excessive need to numb oneself through the use of drugs and/or alcohol, to stay excessively busy, to engage in indiscriminate sex, to spend beyond one's means, or any compulsive behaviors

A common symptom when one is overwhelmed, depleted, and burned out is depression. There are many types of depression with varying causes and origins. Some forms of depression are situational, meaning they are brought on by traumatic or chronically stressful situations, grief and loss, or by the manifestation of compassion fatigue. Other causes of depression are chemical and typically involve a genetic predisposition. Also, trauma experienced during childhood can be hardwired into a child's nervous system; this type of trauma can continue to affect the individual throughout adulthood unless and until it is identified and worked on. Childhood trauma and ongoing stress, combined with certain temperaments, personality types, and environmental components, create an even higher risk of developing compassion fatigue.

The Impact of Chronic Suffering

When some emotional symptoms of compassion fatigue, such as depression, sadness, and apathy, become chronic and still go unattended, the results can be physically devastating. Cardiologist Nieca Goldberg, author of *The Complete Guide to Women's Health* (2009), wrote about how emotions affect physical health. Trauma and loss decrease immune system functioning, causing people to become ill far more frequently than under normal circumstances, especially when the trauma and loss continue over a long period.

According to Karen W. Saakvitne and Laurie Anne Pearlman, professionals who regularly deal with trauma can have difficulty finding a sense of inner balance and often feel less grounded than others. They point out that "their feelings may seem overwhelming: they can have crying jags or eruptions of anger. They can become intolerant or frustrated, unbearably anxious, or chronically unable to experience pleasure. Some, overwhelmed by the trauma of others, shut down emotionally and feel numb, hard, distant, or depersonalized" (Saakvitne and Pearlman 1996, 34).

Denial and Compassion Fatigue

Remember that there is much denial surrounding compassion fatigue, which can affect your ability to recognize it in yourself and seek the help you may need. It's important to remember that one of the most harmful things you can do to yourself is to ignore your own negative or painful feelings and act as if they do not exist. This kind of incongruence between your emotions and your conscious mind aids no one—not you, not your clients, your patients, your family, or your friends. Compassion fatigue has detrimental effects in both your professional and personal life.

Remember that life is all about choices, and you have the power to make choices that will benefit you and help keep your life in balance. You can follow your dreams and enjoy your successes by accessing that inner balance. If you find yourself constantly overwhelmed by your life, you must strive to regain your balance physically, mentally, emotionally, and spiritually and work toward returning to a state of equilibrium. Doing this can prevent being caught in the web of compassion fatigue.

The Effects of Compassion Fatigue on Personal Life

When our sense of responsibility, care, and concern for those we wish to help exceeds our care and concern for ourselves, we are out of balance. When we are out of balance, our family life is likely out of balance. As a result, family members suffer.

Veterinary caregivers suffering from compassion fatigue often end up forfeiting their personal relationships. They sometimes end up in extramarital affairs or may engage in drug and alcohol abuse, which profoundly impacts family members. They can become depressed, anxious, and paranoid. They sometimes lose their internships or residencies, or even their homes. They may end up being arrested, or they may fight with their fellow employees, spouse, and children.

I have worked with many caregivers who needed help battling compassion fatigue. One very bright young veterinarian turned to indiscriminate sex for comfort; tragically, she ended up with AIDS and then lost her marriage. Another professional, a very gifted technician, lost his job because of the vast amounts of alcohol he consumed to numb himself to the horrific images that plagued him. His alcohol consumption, in turn, led to problems with his fellow employees, habitual tardiness, unexplained absences, conflicts with his boss, lying, DUI arrests, and ultimately, termination of his job and the end of his career in veterinary practice.

Another veterinary professional destroyed her family by having an extramarital affair. She not only lost her husband, whom she loved, but also

Compassion Fatigue Self-Assessment

The Professional Quality of Life Scale (ProQOL): Compassion Satisfaction and Compassion Fatigue, created by Dr. Beth Hudnall Stamm, appears later in this chapter. (It is also available at proqol.org.) Consider completing this assessment not just once but regularly. Scoring information appears below the scale. There are no right or wrong answers; the purpose of the scale is to measure your level of compassion fatigue.

Remember, compassion fatigue is a term, not a disease! It is a label to help us identify where we may benefit from healthy changes in our lives. Having a high score does not mean you are in trouble. A high score may mean that there are a number of issues related to your stress that warrant your attention. There is no need for alarm, only awareness. The scores don't matter. What matters are the items on the test that concern you. When you're done with all the scoring, go back through and look for the compassion fatigue items that create stress for you and circle them. Then, use that information to make changes in your life.

had to share custody of her children with him. On more than one occasion, I have worked with veterinary professionals who ended up stealing. These were incredibly self-destructive acts that screamed out for help and attention. Front-office veterinary staff members frequently come to the brink of walking off the job because they have reached their limit; they cannot stand the idea of dealing with one more angry client.

In one case, an intern and a technician fell in love at one of the practices where I consulted, and the relationship seemed to be a perfect match until compassion fatigue destroyed it. She was a beautiful and bright doctor; he was handsome and charming. After her internship ended and she had to be out in "the real world," their relationship could not withstand the pressure she was under. As he put it, she became increasingly distant and "emotionally unreachable," and she agreed. He was hurt that she seemed to have little or no time for him, and although he had stated his concern many times, she did not attempt to rectify the situation. They split up, and she was devastated.

The stories are many and varied, but they have one thing in common: they are all sad and needless. All of these people could have been saved if only they had been proactive in their self-care and sought the support they needed and deserved.

Many people are uncomfortable confronting their emotions and prefer avoiding them, preventing them from dealing with their issues. We are capable of numbing ourselves to our true feelings, but numbing is highly detrimental to our emotional well-being. We must be able to confront our pain and trauma to heal from them. Suppressing our emotions can be much easier, at least in the moment, than dealing with them, but the price we pay for this in the long term is huge.

Distracting yourself from your worries is not the same as numbing yourself: it is normal to seek out distractions to cope with painful emotions temporarily. But numbing yourself stops you from confronting your issues and keeps you from attaining the healing and resolution you deserve.

Although it may be tempting to turn to numbing things, such as alcohol, drugs, shopping, eating, sex, or television, these substitutes offer no real path to healing. Instead, they can become sources of even more difficulties and losses in our lives: failures of relationships, careers, and even the sense of your own identity and self-esteem. It's not worth it. Numbing reduces the quality of your life and blocks your awareness of a deeper need.

On the other hand, activities that ground you and help you feel connected will help you with your sense of balance in life. Doing at least some of these

Professional Quality of Life Scale (ProQOL)

Compassion Satisfaction and Compassion Fatigue

ProQOL Version 5 (2010)

When you [help] people, you have direct contact with their lives. As you may have found, your compassion for those you [help] can positively and negatively affect you. Below are some questions about your experiences, both positive and negative, as a [veterinary professional]. Consider each of the following questions about you and your current work situation. Select the number that honestly reflects how frequently you experienced these things in the *last 30 days.*

1 = Never 2 = Rarely 3 = Sometimes 4 = Often 5 = Very often

___ 1. I am happy.

___ 2. I am preoccupied with more than one person I [help].

___ 3. I get satisfaction from being able to [help] people.

___ 4. I feel connected to others.

___ 5. I jump or am startled by unexpected sounds.

___ 6. I feel invigorated after working with those I [help].

___ 7. I find it difficult to separate my personal life from my life as a [veterinary professional].

___ 8. I am not as productive at work because I am losing sleep over traumatic experiences of a person I [help].

___ 9. I think I might have been affected by the traumatic stress of those I [help].

___ 10. I feel trapped by my job as a [veterinary professional].

___ 11. Because of my [helping], I have felt "on edge" about various things.

___ 12. I like my work as a [veterinary professional].

___ 13. I feel depressed because of the traumatic experiences of the people I [help].

___ 14. I feel like I am experiencing the trauma of someone I have [helped].

___ 15. I have beliefs that sustain me.

___ 16. I am pleased with how I can keep up with [helping] techniques and protocols.

___ 17. I am the person I have always wanted to be.

___ 18. My work makes me feel satisfied.

___ 19. I feel worn out because of my work as a [veterinary professional].

___ 20. I have happy thoughts and feelings about those I [help] and how I could help them.

___ 21. I feel overwhelmed because my [work] load seems endless.

___ 22. I believe I can make a difference through my work.

___ 23. I avoid certain activities or situations because they remind me of the frightening experiences of the people I [help].

___ 24. I am proud of what I can do to [help].

___ 25. Due to my [helping], I have intrusive, frightening thoughts.

___ 26. I feel "bogged down" by the system.

___ 27. I consider myself a "success" as a [veterinary professional].

___ 28. I can't recall important parts of my work with trauma victims.

___ 29. I am a very caring person.

___ 30. I am happy that I chose to do this work.

What Is My Score and What Does It Mean?

In this section, you will score your test so you understand the interpretation for you. To find your score on *each section*, total the questions listed on the left and then find your score in the table on the right of the section.

Compassion Satisfaction Scale

Copy your rating on each of these questions on this table and add them up. When you have added them up, find your score in the table [below].

3. _____	12. _____	18. _____	22. _____	27. _____
6. _____	16. _____	20. _____	24. _____	30. _____

Total: __________

Burnout Scale

On the burnout scale, you will need to take an extra step. Starred items are "reverse scored." If you scored item 1, write a 5 beside it. We ask you to reverse the scores because, scientifically, the measure works better when these questions are asked in a positive way. However, they can tell us more about their negative form—for example, question 1. "I am happy" tells us more about the effects of helping when you are *not* happy, so you reverse the score.

The sum of my compassion questions is	So my score equals	And my compassion satisfaction level is
22 or less	43 or less	Low
Between 23 and 41	Around 50	Average
42 or more	57 or more	High

You wrote	Change to
1	5
2	4
3	3
4	2
5	1

The sum of my burnout:

The sum of my burnout questions is	So my score equals	And my burnout level is
22 or less	43 or less	Low
Between 23 and 41	Around 50	Average
42 or more	57 or more	High

Secondary Traumatic Stress Scale

As you did on compassion satisfaction, copy your rating on each of these questions on this table and add them up. When you have added them up, you can find your score in the table [below].

2. _____ 7. _____ 11. _____ 14. _____ 25. _____

5. _____ 9. _____ 13. _____ 23. _____ 28. _____

Total: __________

The sum of my secondary trauma questions is	So my score equals	And my secondary traumatic stress level is
22 or less	43 or less	Low
Between 23 and 41	Around 50	Average
42 or more	57 or more	High

Your Scores on the ProQOL: Professional Quality of Life Screening

Based on your responses, your personal scores are below. If you have any concerns, you should discuss them with a physical or mental health care professional.

Compassion Satisfaction ___________

Compassion satisfaction is about the pleasure that you derive from being able to do your work well. For example, you may feel like it is a pleasure to help others through your work. You may feel positive about your colleagues, your ability to contribute to the work setting, or even the greater good of society. Higher scores on this scale represent a greater satisfaction related to your ability to be an effective caregiver in your job.

The average score is 50 (standard deviation [SD] = 10; alpha scale reliability = .88). Approximately 25% of people score higher than 57, and approximately 25% score less than 43. If you are in the higher range, you probably derive a good deal of professional satisfaction from your position. If your scores are less than 40, you may either find problems with your job, or there may be some other reason; for example, you might derive your satisfaction from activities other than your job.

Burnout ___________________________

Most people have an intuitive idea of what burnout is. From the research perspective, burnout is one of the elements of compassion fatigue. It is associated with feelings of hopelessness and difficulties in dealing with work or doing your job effectively. These negative feelings usually have a gradual onset. They can reflect the feeling that your efforts make no difference or can be associated with a very high workload or a nonsupportive work environment. Higher scores on this scale mean you are at higher risk of burnout.

The average score on the burnout scale is 50 (SD = 10; alpha scale reliability = .75). Approximately 25% of people score higher than 57, and approximately 25% score less than 43. If your score is less than 18, this reflects positive feelings about your ability to be effective in your work. If you score over 57, you may wish to think about what at work makes you feel like you are ineffective in your position. Your score may reflect your mood; perhaps you were having a "bad day" or need some time off. If the high score persists or reflects other worries, it may be cause for concern.

Secondary Traumatic Stress ____________

The second component of compassion fatigue is secondary traumatic stress. It is about your work-related secondary exposure to significantly or traumatically stressful events. Developing problems due to exposure to others' traumas is rare but happens to many who care for those who have experienced highly or traumatically stressful events. For example, you may repeatedly hear stories about the traumatic things that happen to other people, commonly called vicarious traumatization. You may see or provide treatment to patients who have experienced horrific events. If your work puts you directly in the path of danger due to your work as a soldier or civilian working as military medical personnel, this is not secondary exposure; your exposure is primary. However, this is secondary exposure if you are exposed to others' traumatic events due to your work, such as providing care for casualties or those in a military medical rehabilitation facility. The symptoms of secondary traumatic stress are usually rapid in onset and associated with a particular event. They may include being afraid, having difficulty sleeping, having images of the upsetting event pop into your mind, or avoiding things that remind you of the event.

The average score on this scale is 50 (SD = 10; alpha scale reliability = .81). Approximately 25% of people score less than 43, and approximately 25% score higher than 57. If your score is higher than 57, you should take some time to think about what at work may be frightening to you or whether there is some other reason for the increased score. Although higher scores do not mean that you have a problem, they indicate that you may want to examine how you feel about your work and work environment. You may wish to discuss this with your supervisor, a colleague, or a healthcare professional.

activities daily is essential—and don't forget to laugh! Laughter really is the best medicine.

We have concluded part I of this book. By now, you should know what compassion fatigue is and how it differs from similar conditions, such as stress, burnout, and secondary traumatic stress. You are familiar with common factors in compassion fatigue (including internal and external factors), and you know that attachment and euthanasia both play an essential role in its development. You can understand the symptoms and have a good idea by now whether you are suffering from it. You have gained much knowledge in a few short chapters.

Next, we look at the prevention and treatment of compassion fatigue. By the end of part II, you will know how to find and keep that balance in life to prevent and recover from compassion fatigue.

For the Trainer

After reading chapter 5 and after completing the self-assessment tests, either on your own or as a group, discuss the following:

1. This chapter says, "Remember that life is all about choices, and you have the power to make choices that will benefit you and help keep your life in balance." What do you think "balance" means in this context? Do you think you could make some different choices in your life that would help keep your life balanced? Why or why not?
2. This chapter also says, "On the other hand, activities that ground you and help you feel connected will help you with your sense of balance in life." Have you found activities that help you keep a sense of balance? Share some of these with the group.

PART II

MENTAL HEALTH AND WELL-BEING

6

The Perception of Suffering

We can complain because rose bushes have thorns, or rejoice because thorn bushes have roses.

—ABRAHAM LINCOLN

In cultures of the West, it is not unusual to engage in activities that allow us to feel numb in an attempt to escape from suffering. Suffering is a part of life, but we are taught that we don't need to experience pain and that we should do all we can to escape it. This can end up being attempted in a variety of destructive ways, including suicide.

Avoidance Behaviors

Many of the veterinary professionals with whom I have worked utilize distractions as a way to avoid the heartbreak and ongoing stressors and trauma that can accompany a career in the veterinary or animal-care professions. In other words, they cling to distractions to avoid suffering.

Self-suffering does not diminish when we ignore it. A significant number of people I have spoken to find themselves engaged in constant activity or distractions to avoid having to deal with difficult or painful thoughts and/or emotions. Commonly, people tend to hide from their fear or pain in behaviors such as workaholism, alcohol or drug use, sex, eating/overeating, social media scrolling/cybersurfing, shopping, exercise, constant activity, and constant screen watching. But hiding our pain and pretending it doesn't exist only makes it grow larger. We may be able to temporarily numb ourselves to our suffering, but what happens when we are forced to slow down and be still? Stillness brings insight, and insight is the first step in our ability to stop our suffering.

Human beings suffer in so many ways, but ignoring it simply perpetuates the suffering. I know it can be difficult to admit that you are suffering, given the competitive society surrounding us. Suffering is often seen as a weakness, and it takes much courage to admit that you are experiencing deep pain. But remember this: everyone suffers. Despite how nice or put together one's outer package might appear, we all suffer. We must strive for our truth no matter how painful it might be. To ignore it buries that pain deep within you. That unexpressed negative energy will grow until it can cause emotional pain, as well as physical pain and disease. Some people get to the point that they don't recognize themselves anymore. To avoid these outcomes, we must tell ourselves the truth about our suffering while we surround ourselves with loving-kindness, the way we do so easily for everyone else.

People who have been traumatized often suffer for years following the trauma. A former veterinary technician I worked with would sabotage herself whenever she came close to finding her way free from her trauma. While in her early forties, she sadly lost her mother, followed a year later by her father, and two years after that, her beloved dog passed. She felt victimized for twelve years. She continually questioned why she had to endure so much loss and what she did to deserve it. She suffered daily because she had not come to terms with her past losses. She suffered because, rather than finding the gifts in the present moment, she chose to dwell in the pain from the past. If we can accept how things are, we will maintain the ability to find happiness. We have no control over what life brings us, but we can control how we deal with it.

Sadly, many people don't believe they are entitled to joy or happiness. Veterinary and animal-care professionals tend to be very hard on themselves. They set standards for themselves far above what they set for everyone else. One of the greatest veterinary technicians I've ever known is horribly hard on herself. She is always the first to jump in and help an animal or another human being. She was one of the first volunteers assisting animals and people in the aftermath of Hurricane Katrina. She fights for others, but sadly, she doesn't appear to have an ounce of loving-kindness for herself. After knowing this incredible woman for many years, I feel confident enough to say she has no self-compassion. She is extremely compassionate to others but will never take a stand for herself. This brilliant, sensitive, and kind person suffers from chronic depression, anxiety, and low self-esteem. Though she has a stellar work ethic, she has no social life and has never experienced a long-term relationship. She beats herself up if she even thinks she made a mistake, which only perpetuates the cycle of negativity. It's horrible to witness someone who defines herself not by the kindness and care she constantly gives to others but rather by those few times when she felt that she should have done more, even if it was not within her control to do so.

Our greatest struggles can make us stronger and teach us who we truly are. Our toughest challenges often teach us how durable we can be. My technician friend needs to understand that she is not defined by what she did or didn't do in the past. The only thing that matters is how she acts right here, right now. She must learn how to forgive herself and realize that we all make mistakes, and if we choose to, we can learn from them and grow. I wish for her to confront her suffering to understand her need to hold herself to such an impossible standard. Once she realizes the suffering she is causing herself, she can begin to use loving-kindness and self-compassion. With this, she can learn how to let go of her need to be perfect to have self-worth. I want her to know that she is perfect just as she is so she can be happy and at ease.

Cultivating Self-Compassion

> *Self-love, self-respect, self-worth: There's a reason they all start with self. You can't find them in anyone else.*
>
> —ROB LIANO

Everyone deserves a fulfilling life with minimal suffering. However, to have this, caregiving veterinary professionals and animal-care specialists must commit to consistent self-care, including being completely honest with themselves and asking for help when needed. A large part of self-care comes from a strong sense of self-knowledge; knowing yourself well is pivotal in developing effective coping skills, resiliency, mindful communication skills, and overall self-care.

Finding a Place of Rest

In Frank Ostaseski's brilliant book *The Five Invitations: What the Living Can Learn from the Dying* (2017), he speaks of five principles that allow us to live our lives fully and find a place of rest in the middle of things. Without changing our lives or circumstances, Ostaseski says we can find that place of rest within ourselves. It is amazing to see what being kind to ourselves can do for the quality of our lives. Self-compassion can liberate us daily.

In our competitive Western culture, we commonly permit ourselves to rest only after we have accomplished everything else we have told ourselves we must do on that day. Our love for others should be no different from the love and compassion we hold for ourselves. If your elderly parents were tired, you would encourage them to rest. If your children were hungry, you would feed them. And yet many adults don't feed themselves. It is common for me to see veterinary and animal-care professionals ignore feelings of hunger or exhaustion as they "power through" their lives day after day.

I grew up in California, surrounded by typical Western values, so I never learned how to rest. Until recently, I believed that rest held no value because it was unproductive. While still a child in elementary school, I had a conversation with my beloved father. He was returning home from work early one evening and noticed me high up in the branches of a walnut tree in our front yard. He inquired why I was up there, and I responded that I loved how it felt. He asked me whether my homework, pet-related chores, and piano practice were completed, and I proudly assured him that all had been done. "What about the vocabulary words I gave you for this week?" he inquired, and I was pleased to tell him that I had memorized the list the day prior. My father said that while he was pleased that I had taken care of all my responsibilities, resting in a tree or anywhere else was not very constructive behavior, and he was sure we could find me an activity of greater value. I grew up associating resting with laziness.

Embracing Self-Compassion for Healing and Growth

Much suffering is caused when things don't go how we want or expect them to. Many wonderful people constantly play an internal recording of the painful things that have happened to them. They concentrate only on the bad or painful experiences of their lives, giving little thought to all the gifts they have received or all the good things they have done for others. Many express that they don't have enough to be lovable. They say that they don't have a good enough education, home, job, relationship, or car; or that they are not smart enough, attractive enough, fit enough, courageous enough, or lovable enough to ever be successful. It's tragic to watch people continually criticize and blame themselves because of their perception of their inadequacies. I've seen many whose own inner critic leaves them feeling worthless over and over again, regardless of all the good they have done.

We must learn to be kind and compassionate toward ourselves, just as we strive to be with everyone else. We must learn to forgive ourselves when we think we messed up. No matter how much good they do in this world for others, the majority of animal-care professionals I have worked with believe they are never good enough. Instead of the thousands they have saved, their thoughts often go to those they could not help, and they typically beat themselves up for it over and over again.

We can see the best in others and ourselves by changing what we view as perfection. Don't let the few cases that didn't go your way blind you to the multiple cases that did. We may have to change how we view success to learn to love and acknowledge ourselves precisely as we are.

Be like the animals you live and work with and practice self-compassion. I realize that having compassion and kindness for yourself is challenging in our competitive culture. Still, to maintain our compassion for other beings and to

Case Study | Betty

Our strong drive to "prove ourselves" stems from being raised in a competitive society. How we regard ourselves tends to be associated with how we perform. Our children should understand that our love for them is without conditions. Betty, a brilliant specialist I worked with, came to me for compassion fatigue support, and it quickly became apparent that she was unduly harsh on herself. She held herself to a standard that allowed no room for anything less than perfection. It was difficult to listen to the horrible things she would say about herself when she felt she had let down a patient, a client, or a loved one. During our third session, while discussing the importance of self-care, Betty revealed that she always slept with her eyes open and that it was a bit disconcerting for her husband the first few times they spent the night together. When I inquired why she thought she did that, Betty responded that she never felt safe. In a subsequent session, Betty revealed that as a child, if she didn't have the highest grade possible on every school exam, when her father returned home late at night, he would go into her room to awaken her and hit her with a strap. By the time she was in the fourth grade, Betty had stopped being able to close her eyes when she would finally fall asleep.

connect with them in a way that allows us to awaken to what they need, we must start with ourselves.

Thupten Jinpa, PhD, a Buddhist scholar and the primary English translator to the Dalai Lama since 1985, speaks of the need for us to have self-acceptance and to be a friend to ourselves. He says self-compassion "asks us to bring a genuine sense of caring to our experience and respond to it with understanding, acceptance, and kindness. This is what we do when we respond compassionately to the needs and suffering of a loved one—nothing more, nothing mysterious" (Jinpa 2015, 46). In Eastern countries, self-image is high, he says, and confidence is low. In the West, on the other hand, Dr. Jinpa says that confidence is high while self-compassion is low. In her excellent book *Self-Compassion: Stop Beating Yourself Up and Leave Insecurity Behind*, Kristin Neff speaks about how, in our society, we must feel that we are special and above average to feel worthy. In her self-compassion exercises, Neff begins by asking us to treat ourselves as we would a good friend who was struggling (Neff 2015).

We all have challenges. Many people believe they could be happy if they changed the circumstances in their lives. From what I have seen, it doesn't work that way. I have often witnessed clients work hard to change something about their lives, but the moment they accomplish their goal, they self-sabotage because their vision of themselves does not match their success. In our culture, we most often need to learn how to treat ourselves with kindness. How much do we appreciate someone whom we are constantly trying to fix?

Whenever animal caregivers, from veterinary specialists to shelter workers, speak in a self-degrading manner, I ask them to please restate the sentence while replacing the negative with at least one positive thing about themselves. By being honest and real, we see that we all make the same mistakes, which is a part of our shared humanity. Stop thinking that you are the only one who has messed up; we are human—it's what we do!

Tsenzhab Serkong Rinpoche II, considered one of the most valid Buddhist teachers of the new generation by His Holiness, the Dalai Lama, says that compassion is not only for others; it always includes yourself as well (Rinpoche 2015). To continue to help others, I know I must take good care of myself. Mother Teresa used to tell us to "love until it hurts," which she did, and which I know animal-care professionals can relate to. However, she didn't add to love and be kind to yourself so that you can continue to love others. Helping other beings feels good, but we cannot continue doing it if we do not care for ourselves. Compassion toward others can be furthered only by being compassionate toward ourselves.

A mentor of mine mentioned that unless I learned to care for and be compassionate toward myself, I would eventually be unable to take care of others. Those words woke me up to the importance of self-care and self-compassion. The other gift of learning to be compassionate toward ourselves is that it furthers our ability to be compassionate toward others. Many veterinary professionals have a hard time cultivating compassion for themselves. They are commonly their own harshest critics.

For the Trainer

After reading chapter 6, either on your own or as a group, discuss the following:

1. What sort of distractions do you engage in as an attempt to avoid suffering?
2. What are a few ways that you can surround yourself with loving-kindness?
3. Do you hold yourself to a nearly impossible standard? Why or why not?
4. Do you think you have all you need to be a joyful and well-functioning adult? Why or why not?
5. How might you be more compassionate toward yourself?
6. Part of staying in balance is rest. How do you plan to get more in touch with nature's rhythm and get the rest you need?

7

Hospice and Palliative Care Professionals

Knowing yourself is the beginning of wisdom.

—ARISTOTLE

Working with the dying and the families of the dying is among the most gut-wrenchingly painful work one can do, but it is also among the greatest of honors. Those accompanying other beings through the end of their lives face no easy task as they follow their goal, which is the same goal that many in the animal-care professions share: alleviating suffering.

Veterinary hospice and palliative care professionals often form deep relationships with the pets and the families of the pets they treat. Such professionals therefore often experience a deep sense of compounded grief when a pet in their care dies. Compounded grief is caused by cumulative losses appearing within a short period. Hospice and palliative care professionals must continually deal with compounded, ongoing loss and must therefore learn to protect themselves from its potentially detrimental effects. Many attempt to use their professional boundaries as protection against surrendering to the ongoing pain and lack of a well-balanced life. We are quickly shown, however, that professional boundaries are sadly not enough in the battle against compassion fatigue.

Certain factors can influence your experience of grief and loss, most of which revolve around intensity. The intensity of the relationship determines how intense the grief will be. Self-awareness is vital in helping you understand your emotions instead of being overwhelmed by them. Recognizing your strengths and weaknesses and knowing why you react the way you do to certain emotions will help you manage them. Refer to the list of the symptoms of compassion fatigue in chapter 5 and see how many apply to you.

Self-Care and Mindfulness

Self-care strategies and mindfulness are both crucial for maintaining a good quality of life as hospice or palliative care professionals. Along with the many losses, the heightened emotionality, and the ongoing psychological challenges, witnessing the suffering of others is often highly traumatic. Through consistent self-care, you can work in the face of trauma and suffering while maintaining your health physically, emotionally, mentally, and spiritually. Self-care requires discipline and practice; however, by committing to it, you can bring the best of yourself to your patients, clients, coworkers, friends, loved ones, and most of all, to yourself.

Mindfulness is being fully aware of your present situation—your thoughts, perceptions, and feelings—moment by moment. By staying in the present, there is no possibility of dwelling in the past, nor is there the possibility of becoming anxious about the future and what might or might not happen. The past is any moment before the present one, and the future is any moment after it.

Mindfulness may at first seem counterintuitive, as veterinary hospice and palliative care revolve around death, dying, and the alleviation of suffering. As such, these compassionate people cannot help but suffer as well. The trick is to be able to show up fully every day, even for your own suffering. Although it may not sound like it, mindfulness is really quite simple, but it does require practice. It involves observing ourselves and the situation, in the present moment, without judgment, and gently refocusing ourselves if we find our mind has drifted away.

A consistent mindfulness practice improves the quality of our lives and relationships while allowing us the space to respond consistently to situations rather than react to them. Not only does mindfulness practice allow us to feel calm, it also increases our awareness. It will enable us to intercept our minds if we notice we dwell on negative thoughts or ruminate on the past or future. Mindfulness also helps us build resilience, allowing us to recover rapidly from adversity or difficult situations. Through practicing mindfulness, I hope you will be able to face the enormous challenges of working with the dying in a far more self-compassionate way. More in-depth information on mindfulness can be found in chapter 9.

Mirror Neurons

When we are calm, it tends to calm those around us. As noted in chapter 2, this is possible because of the mirror neurons in our brain's premotor cortex. Mirror neurons are the reason we can feel empathy for others, which of course is imperative and highly beneficial to our patients and their families, as well as to our coworkers, friends, and loved ones. Both humans and primates have mirror neurons, which allow us to observe the behavior of another being while feeling as if we are doing the same action (Siegel 2020). For example, I was walking years ago when I saw a child on a bike fall and slide on the hot pavement. When I helped him up, his knees were bleeding, and when I saw that, my own knees felt as if they were also torn and bleeding. In other words, both action execution and action observation can elicit the same results.

Several years ago, I first spoke about the importance of mirror neurons at a veterinary conference sponsored by Dr. Mona Rosenberg, a brilliant veterinary oncologist and founder of the Veterinary Cancer Group and City of Angels Veterinary Specialty Center. I was lecturing about the self-care benefits of guided imagery and how the body does not discriminate between what is real and what is perceived or imagined. This is important when working with the families of hospice and palliative care patients, as it offers one more way to relate to what they are experiencing. It also provides us with further options in self-care. For more information, see chapter 18, "Coping: The Importance of Self Care."

Loving-Kindness

During my time in India, I gratefully learned about mindfulness meditation and loving-kindness meditation, which help us comfort ourselves during painful or difficult times. Remember that words have an enormous influence on how we feel about ourselves. The words we tell ourselves are vitally important, whether spoken or not. We suffer when we say or even think unkind things about ourselves. The Buddhist tradition teaches that loving and kind phrases can be particularly helpful in creating self-kindness.

Loving-kindness teaches us how to be gentler with ourselves. Without expectations, try repeating the following at least once a day:

May I be happy
May I be free from suffering
May I be free from sorrow
May I love myself as I am

In time, you can add the following if you wish:

May all beings be happy
May all beings be free from suffering
May all beings be free from sorrow
May all beings love themselves as they are

And remember, when painful feelings pull you away from the present moment, allow your breath to gently bring you back. Allow your breath to be your connection back to yourself, in the present moment, here and now. *Sama vritti* pranayama is a yogic practice that increases a sense of calm while decreasing stress. "Sama vritti" means equal breathing, and it can be very effective in helping us deal with stressful or painful situations. Try this exercise: sitting or lying in a comfortable position, gently close your eyes and begin noticing your breath. Inhale through your nose for a slow count of five and then exhale through your nose again for a slow count of five. Do this five times and increase when you are comfortable.

For the Trainer

After reading chapter 7, either on your own or as a group, discuss the following:

1. How do you take care of yourself so you can face the enormous challenges of working with those suffering or dying?
2. Which of your strengths help you deal with the ongoing traumatic situations you encounter in your career as an animal-care professional?
3. Which of your weaknesses impede you in your career?
4. How do you think being able to stop your negative thoughts, particularly about yourself, and not ruminating about something that happened or something you saw or heard in the past might help you in the work you do? How about in your personal relationships?

8

How We Think

Carefully watch your thoughts for they become your words.

—MAHATMA GANDHI

More than anything else, our thoughts determine how we feel. How and what we think affects our health, well-being, and sense of comfort and safety. Of the many veterinary and animal-care professionals who have sat before me, those who typically have a positive outlook on life tend to move through life's challenges faster. And they tend to heal more quickly when recovering from compassion fatigue, grief, depression, trauma, and anxiety than those who think negatively. People with a pessimistic outlook tend to stay stuck in their self-defeating thoughts and subsequent feelings of sadness, loneliness, anger, envy, resentment, and victimization. It's impossible to cultivate a sense of well-being if you constantly remind yourself of why you don't deserve to be happy. Negative thinkers tend to think of only those things that can go wrong and give little attention when something good happens. Yet a sense of well-being has a strong connection to happiness and satisfaction in life.

The Power of Thoughts

We must first take power over our own thoughts to take power over our lives. In his groundbreaking book *The Power of Positive Thinking: A Practical Guide to Mastering the Problems of Everyday Living,* Norman Vincent Peale wrote that people commonly give up on their power by thinking that they don't have any. Peale pointed out that people who consistently think negatively are often unaware of when something positive happens, as they are focused only on things that didn't go right or might not go right in the future (Peale 1952). It can sometimes seem as if negative thinkers are afraid to be happy. An amazing veterinary professional I know is one such individual. He will not allow himself to own any of his wins or even enjoy the beauty of a peaceful moment because he is constantly telling himself how much better he could have done or that something bad is simply waiting right around the corner.

People who have always tended to think negatively seem to concentrate exclusively on why they won't do well or won't be successful, even when there have been positive changes in their lives. I sadly watch as they take away their ability to experience a sense of joy, happiness, or pride in their accomplishments. Instead, they choose to remain stuck in their negative thought patterns. Here is an exercise you can try: when you judge yourself harshly, imagine someone who loves you and change your thoughts to what their thoughts and words of encouragement would be. This way, you can turn off your inner critic and make it easier to accept praise from yourself.

Knowing that life contains both good and bad moments and being able to stay present in any situation are of great importance when working in any caregiving position. Developing equanimity—accepting both the good and the bad while maintaining composure—allows our minds to stay calm and level-headed, which is better for our overall well-being. Matthieu Ricard, a world-renowned Buddhist monk and writer, speaks of incredible deviations in the definitions of happiness. Ricard believes simply that how we think defines how we feel. He has indicated that how we think underlies all emotional states, and therefore a sense of well-being is not about a momentary sense of peacefulness or fulfillment (Ricard 2012).

Most people, especially in Western countries, seek happiness outside themselves. It's not uncommon for people to say they will be happy once they complete their internship, get a home of their own, find a new job, begin a relationship, or bring in a certain amount of income. Yet these thoughts offer only temporary delusions of happiness—once attained, yet another goal generally replaces them. This means that happiness is never really achieved. If you instead consider that thinking is what defines happiness, you can begin to reframe happiness as something that comes from inside yourself. This mindful thinking gives us the gift of the present moment. When we think mindfully, we are not stuck in regrets about the past or filled with anxiety over what will or won't happen in the future.

Mindfulness

I first heard about the concept of mindfulness from the Buddhist monk and Zen master Thich Nhat Hanh in his life-altering book *The Miracle of Mindfulness: An Introduction to the Practice of Meditation*. The practice of mindfulness encourages a calm and relaxed way of moving through life that doesn't focus on past or future issues. Nhat Hanh suggests starting by setting aside one day a week to practice being mindful (Nhat Hanh 1975). As a caregiver dealing with the trauma of others daily, I found this exercise to be a welcome relief. When starting out, I took one day per week to complete all my usual tasks in a slower, more thoughtful way, all the while concentrating on my breath. At first it was difficult, and I had to keep reminding myself to come back to my breath. But as I practiced, it became easier, and I can now move through each day more mindfully aware of the present moment. I was always known for being an expert at multitasking, but I am no longer proud of that. Through these teachings and my practice of mindfulness, I have learned how to throw myself fully into the present moment and focus on bad and good situations, conversations, and tasks, no matter how small. Doing so has given me a sense of calm, appreciation, full presence, and deep connection.

For the Trainer

After reading chapter 8, either on your own or as a group, discuss the following:

1. Do you tend to think about all the things that could go wrong in your personal or professional life (or both)? Why or why not?
2. Do you celebrate the things you feel you did well? Why or why not?
3. What are some ways you can stay open to the good things in life?

9

The Dangers of Social Media

If you think you are too small to make a difference, try sleeping with a mosquito.

—THE DALAI LAMA

Social media continually evolves, and its use has increased dramatically in the last decade. Social media allows people from all over the world to communicate with one another. Its primary limitation, however, is that it cannot guarantee reliability. Authors offering veterinary practice advice or other information often need to be discovered.

Social Media Risks

Because of the high probability of incorrect information being shared on social media, it can negatively affect the careers of veterinary and animal-care professionals. This is possible primarily because anyone can write anything on social media, true or not. It is therefore easy to understand how simply boundaries can be eschewed and legal issues increased, not to mention the detriment to one's professional image.

Another danger related to social media is unprofessional posts that can reflect negatively on veterinarians or animal-care professionals and organizations. Social media conveys information about people's private lives and their values through their followers and friends, the content or photos they post, and the groups they belong to. Most employers now regularly search social networking sites when considering someone for a job, an internship, a residency program, or admission to a professional program.

If veterinary or animal-care professionals use social media wisely, it can effectively promote their practice and themselves. However, when used carelessly, social media can prove to be dangerous and even deadly. We all must remember that once something is posted online, regardless of privacy settings, it may be accessible forever. To protect ourselves, we must always maintain the highest standards of professionalism and be thoughtful about what we choose to post.

Cyberbullying

In 2014, largely as a result of cyberbullying, the veterinary profession lost a brilliant veterinarian, Dr. Shirley Koshi. Dr. Koshi took her own life in large part because of lies that were posted about her on social media and the public harassment that followed. Some of her colleagues told me that Dr. Koshi helped a woman who was homeless and living in the Bronx. They said the woman brought her cat into the veterinary office, where she examined him. The cat needed surgery, but knowing that the woman had no money, she offered to do the surgery for free. The two agreed that after the cat recovered, he would live at the veterinary practice and the woman would be welcome to visit him as much as she liked during business hours.

Dr. Koshi's colleagues further said that it was nearly two years before the woman returned to the veterinary practice again. When she did, she intended to take the cat with her. I was told that she started to demand loudly that the cat be returned to her. The kindly veterinarian inquired and learned that the woman was still living on the streets and dealing with extreme elements. When Dr. Koshi gently explained that it would be in the cat's best interest to allow him to continue to live at the hospital and that she could still visit him whenever she liked, the woman became infuriated and started screaming obscenities, accusations, and threats at the veterinarian and her staff. This client began posting horrible lies about her and her practice on social media. As a result, the veterinarian began losing clients and a large part of her income until she was finally forced to close her practice. Not long after that, we were given the heartbreaking news that this beautiful being had taken her own life. A study by the American Veterinary Medical Association tragically revealed that one in five veterinarians had been cyberbullied or knew of a colleague who had been (AVMA 2023). Many of these veterinary professionals are also threatened (Bekiari and Pachi 2017).

I have witnessed too many times how manipulative people can become when getting what they want takes precedence over their own integrity. I remember a time when I was called in by one of my favorite specialty practice owners who was having difficulty dealing with one such client. The client was vicious to the staff members and the specialist working on her dog's case. The practice manager called in the practice owner, who came in immediately. This amazing woman is among the kindest and most compassionate people I've ever known. She called me in when she could make no headway with this client.

After the appropriate introductions, the client began telling us why she felt she should not have to pay for the services her dog had already received. She was belligerent and threatening, and it took some time to calm her down. We had to discount her bill significantly and promise her a few complimentary services. With that, she finally turned it around and, instead of verbally attacking us, began complimenting the entire veterinary team. We told her we would get the certificates for the complimentary services, and she thanked us profusely as we left the room. Walking down the hall, we passed the employee break room, where one of the technicians was having lunch. He called us over and asked how it was going with the client. When we explained that she had calmed down and was actually expressing appreciation, he laughed and said, "That's hilarious." He showed us on his phone that the moment the door had shut behind us, the woman had posted a review on Yelp in an attempt to destroy the reputation of this superb veterinarian. The most challenging part of this whole scenario was that we had to walk back into the treatment room with gift certificates in hand and act as if we didn't know what she had just posted online. This trend has become a huge concern of mine.

For the Trainer

After reading chapter 9, either on your own or as a group, discuss the following:

1. How do you protect yourself when it comes to social media?
2. How would you handle cyberbullying?
3. How might you adjust your perception of cyberbullying?

10

The Difference Between Ethics Fatigue, Moral Fatigue, and Compassion Fatigue

There can be no greater gift than that of giving one's time and energy to help others without expecting anything in return.

—NELSON MANDELA

Ethics Fatigue

Ethics fatigue in the animal-care field results from feeling forced to do things that we consider ethically reprehensible. It is the emotional distress and fatigue of not being able to act on what we believe is the correct and compassionate thing to do, especially when we have to do so repeatedly. Going against our beliefs and doing something immoral or wrong is extremely difficult and emotionally taxing. It is a horrible conflict between what we feel is right and what we must do to stay employed.

Among those who feel ethically helpless, it's easy to understand why we often hear comments such as "I had no choice, I had to do it," or "No one else seems to care, why should I?" These veterinary professionals are trying to justify something that left them feeling guilty, and in many cases, ashamed.

Sonnya Dennis, DVM, DABVP, introduced the term "ethics exhaustion" to describe the feeling of fatigue, emotional strain, and loss of motivation to consistently act in a manner that aligns with your ethical principles (Lengyel 2018). According to Dr. Dennis, "Ethics exhaustion is not a decline in compassion. Instead, it occurs when you are repeatedly unable to act in a compassionate and caring way due to various constraints, to the point where you stop making the effort or caring" (Lengyel 2018).

The most difficult ethical dilemmas I'm aware of involved euthanasia of perfectly healthy pets regardless of how young and healthy they were. It's difficult to listen to. I can't imagine how devastating it must be to feel forced to engage in it.

Unfortunately, there has been a significant increase in ethics fatigue cases over the last eight to ten years. This increase is commonly blamed on the number of corporate takeovers. Many in the veterinary profession now feel as though their hands are tied regarding how much they can help a particular pet. Many have expressed that the bottom line is the only thing that seems to matter now, taking precedence over everything else. People in veterinary specialty medicine who have been practicing for many years have shared with me that in the past, they were able to appeal to upper management to set up payment plans for clients who could not otherwise afford treatment. Many feel they are prevented from advocating for the pet and are barred from providing correct and compassionate care. Often, feelings of depression and anger arise in such situations. Forced to act contrary to their belief system, they feel emotionally exhausted, which has an impact on compassion fatigue.

Moral Fatigue

Moral fatigue is a state of emotional exhaustion and detachment that can occur when a person is repeatedly exposed to morally difficult situations. In veterinary medicine, this could include conditions in which a veterinarian must make difficult decisions about patient care, such as when to euthanize an animal. Moral fatigue can lead to feelings of cynicism, apathy, and burnout.

Moral fatigue is to be expected in veterinary and animal-care professionals, who tend to have more than their share of ongoing moral conflicts. "Ethically challenging situations (ECS) are common in veterinary settings and can lead to moral stress" (Quain et al. 2021). When veterinarians' duties to their patients are uncertain and are being influenced by management, the cultural climate of their work gets altered. For instance, a client may bring in a perfectly healthy young dog for euthanasia because the client was "having family in for the holidays" and didn't "want to have to deal with the dog." In such disgusting and painful situations, professionals become increasingly depressed and exhausted. I have known a few who left practices to find groups instead or start practices that shared their morals.

In a cognitive sense, moral fatigue is related to compassion fatigue in professionals who are constantly exposed to traumatic situations. According to Charles R. Figley, two categories of moral suffering lead to traumatization: moral distress emanating from morally conflicted cases, and moral injury (Figley 2015). Moral distress regularly occurs when veterinary or animal-care professionals recognize the correct way to help an animal, but they cannot pursue it because of the policies of their management team.

Learned Helplessness

Ethics fatigue and moral fatigue can contribute to and exist simultaneously with compassion fatigue. In fact, both can contribute to the development of compassion fatigue and learned helplessness. Learned helplessness is a condition where people feel powerless, which often stems from dealing with continual traumatic events or a consistent failure to achieve in a way they find morally acceptable. Additionally, it is believed to be a common underlying cause of depression. Having to suppress how they feel and go along with what they believe is wrong or immoral can cause animal-care professionals to say things like "I had no choice" and "Why should I care when nobody else does?" Their exhaustion, combined with emotional suffering, should be of great concern to all practice owners and managers.

Recognizing and Alleviating Ethics and Moral Fatigue

Veterinary professionals typically seek out ways to enhance the lives of pets and their families. The moment a family receives a terminal diagnosis regarding their beloved pet, they begin grieving and find themselves in a very vulnerable state. At such times, pet families commonly turn to their veterinary professionals for comfort, knowledge, and hope. The challenge is that animal professionals often neglect and sacrifice their own needs to help others.

For veterinary professionals, ethical concerns have always included making proper diagnoses and treatment plans for their patients, often at a moment's notice in emergent situations, which allow no room for mistakes. Being able to continue doing this, sometimes several times a day, requires ongoing self-care. But in time, the compounding of all these difficult decisions can cause compassion to lessen, especially when one is suffering from compassion fatigue and dealing with ethics fatigue simultaneously.

Combined, these disorders can steal our ability to feel compassion or empathy for others. Both compassion fatigue and ethics fatigue result from working in a profession that requires compassion but forces professionals to deal with the continual trauma, suffering, and deaths of pets, along with the emotional suffering of pet owners who cannot afford the ever-rising costs of veterinary medicine. So, veterinary and animal-care professionals are at high risk for developing these disorders because of the difficult decisions they have to make. The vast amount of physical, emotional, financial, and mental stress in the veterinary profession cannot be ignored. This stress is compounded when many caregivers are forced to deal with several ethical concerns daily. Self-care can be effective at helping prevent compassion fatigue and ethics fatigue, but such professionals must first deal with any unresolved trauma or grief from their past.

I am concerned about the impact these moral conflicts have on veterinary and other animal-care professionals. Veterinary practice has changed significantly over time, becoming far less personal and far more corporate. Making sure that the treatment is not worse than the disease, paying attention to the quality of life of pets and the needs of pet families, and being proactive about self-care should be the primary concerns of all animal-care professionals everywhere.

While presenting a continuing education lecture to veterinarians on compassion fatigue, I had the distinct pleasure of running into a brilliant and dynamic veterinarian. After the lecture, she approached the stage and shared her thoughts on ethics fatigue with the crowd. This incredible woman, Alice Villalobos, DVM, FNAP, brought compassion to cancer care for companion animals and to pet hospice. She also demonstrated a way of looking at patients as individuals with their own needs and sensitivities that need to be honored and respected.

Clients in my pet-loss support groups have often shared that Villalobos is in a class of her own. "She is not afraid to think outside the box and treat each and every pet as an individual, not a number," said Julie, one of her long-time clients. As such, Dr. Villalobos, combined with her extensive and ongoing research, has a comfort level that allows her to explore more than just the most common treatment protocols. She is well known for her success with oncology patients and for the Pawspice Quality of Life Scale she created (Villalobos 2011). This scale has helped thousands of pet owners make the gut-wrenching decision to give their loved ones the peaceful passing they deserve.

When Dr. Villalobos took the stage that evening, she spoke of the need to continue addressing compassion fatigue proactively, considering that ethics fatigue may sneak through just beneath our awareness. Thanks to Dr. Villalobos and her tremendous contributions, ethics fatigue no longer has to go unrecognized within the mechanisms of compassion fatigue.

Dr. Villalobos also spoke about the human-animal bond and how, historically, humans performed the role of the good shepherd, which is a contract humans formed with animals during ancient times. To honor this contract, she teaches that we must allow our pets who are reaching the end of their lives, whose quality of life has begun to decline, and who, without human intervention, will eventually suffer, a "compassionate, quality death," where we are honored to escort them and play witness to their peaceful passing. "Our pets," she said, "rely on us totally as their keepers to help them make that transition."

A common component of compassion fatigue in veterinary-care professionals is the toll that performing frequent euthanasia takes. Dr. Villalobos suggests that veterinary teams try to think of euthanasia in a more favorable light, remembering that the kindness and compassion they offer pets and their families at such a painful time is both a good deed and a blessing.

For the Trainer

After reading chapter 10, either on your own or as a group, discuss the following:

1. What would you do if your employer tried to force you to engage in behavior that you find immoral or wrong?
2. What can you do to feel less powerless and more empowered in your career?
3. Have you dealt with the trauma and grief of your past? If so, how did you do it? Was it helpful?

PART III

CREATING A POSITIVE WORKPLACE CULTURE

11

Alleviating Gossip and Its Potentially Deadly Effects

You are not only responsible for what you say but also for what you do not say.
—MARTIN LUTHER

The most powerful way of changing a negative workplace culture into a positive one is by prohibiting gossip. Gossiping involves saying something untrue, unnecessary, or scandalous about someone else's personal business. Another type of gossiping, backbiting, is a harsher version that involves more slanderous content and more spiteful intent. How many people do you know who are not affected by the gossip aimed at them? Gossip can ruin people's lives and even be the final straw behind the decision to take one's own life. Gossip creates a toxic and unhealthy work atmosphere that feels emotionally unsafe. Many people fear being open and honest about their thoughts and feelings where gossip is allowed to exist.

With all of life's challenges in the veterinary and animal-care professions, management teams can help lessen absenteeism, turnover rates, and the number of employee violations simply by creating a sense of safety with a no-tolerance policy for gossip that is strictly enforced. If we are genuinely concerned, as we should be, about bullying at schools and on social media, we must model and provide work environments where gossip is not tolerated.

Religious and Cultural Principles Related to Gossip

Most religions and cultural traditions have always had rules or teachings on the importance of not gossiping about other people. Most regard talking behind someone's back as something very serious and even dangerous. It is typically among the highest guiding principles of behavior in various traditions. Not speaking ill of another person is included, for example, in the first precepts of Buddhism, under the precept of refraining from incorrect speech.

"Never speaking about the faults of others" or "refraining from speaking about others" and "not committing haphazard talk" are different ways I've heard scholars refer to the importance of not gossiping. We should never take gossip as the truth and never pass it on to someone else. We must be mindful when we speak as well as when we listen. I learned early in life to walk away from the other kids on the playground who were speaking poorly of another child. I still excuse myself in such situations.

The truth is that gossip can ruin people's lives. It commonly tears families and friendships apart. Another great tradition, Judaism, speaks of the importance of not gossiping in the Talmud. This holy book teaches that relaying gossip has the potential to kill three: the one who says it, the one who listens to it, and the person who is the subject of the gossip.

Speaking poorly about another person's shortcomings or behaviors is called *lashon hara* in Hebrew, which means "evil tongue." Thanks to the teachings of Rabbi Israel Meir Kagan (the Chofetz Chaim), there has been increased awareness in the past several decades about the dangers of gossip. His teachings say that one is forbidden not only from speaking gossip but from listening to it as well, "for there can be no gossip if there is no one there to listen" (Finkelman, Berkowitz, and Meir 1995).

The Islamic religion has always banned gossiping and has some well-known quotes about it, including "Gossip dies when it hits a wise person's ears." My favorite is "Who gossips with you, will gossip about you." I taught my children when they were quite young that if a friend of theirs was talking badly about another friend who was not present, then the first friend was probably talking badly about them when they were not around as well. You can only walk away from gossip, change the subject, or, best of all, let the person know that you make it a practice not to listen to gossip and that you will do what you have to do in order not to hear it.

Christianity prohibits gossip, and several Bible passages address it. As an example, James 1:26 says, "Those who consider themselves religious and yet do not keep a tight rein on their tongues deceive themselves, and their religion is worthless." In Leviticus 19:16, we find "Do not go spreading slander among your people. Do not do anything that endangers your neighbor's life." The Catholic church also teaches that gossip typically involves uncharitable or inappropriate conversations about others who are not present. It includes such talk in its treatment of the Eighth Commandment: "You shall not bear false witness against your neighbor." Saint Thomas also included it in his treatise on justice; when referring to gossip, he said, "Since by it, we unjustly harm the reputation of others, for the introduction of errors and variations into the information transmitted."

Why People Gossip

So why do people gossip in the first place? I have noticed that many people who tend to gossip also appear to need attention. Wanting to be the deliverer of information, the one in the know, or the one everyone gathers around at a party or function to hear the latest is a great pull to such individuals. Sometimes the goal is to simply entertain, and sometimes it is an attempt to get closer to others at the expense of another person. Sadly, some people gossip out of anger or jealousy in an effort to destroy another person's life, as we have unfortunately witnessed.

Impact of Gossip

I've also spoken with several veterinary professionals who were having trouble with absenteeism, and management had talked to them about it. When I asked the employees why they thought they were having trouble getting to work, many said they were extremely anxious about having to face constant gossip and backbiting. Several of those people went on medical leave, and many were prescribed antianxiety medications to function.

Techniques for Eliminating Gossip

We need to ask ourselves what our motivation is if we desire to talk poorly about someone who is not present or spread false rumors about them. In Buddhism, it is taught that the value of one's speech depends primarily on the motivation behind it.

If you are ever tempted to speak poorly about someone else, try stopping first and asking yourself what that person's positive attributes are. What is something you like about that person? Think about it: there has to be at least one thing you like or appreciate about them. Next, ask yourself in what ways they might be similar to you. Who knows, instead of causing harm, you may build bridges.

Exercising self-control over our speech is highly admirable. Even greater is the ability to treat all beings with dignity and respect. Doing so allows us to automatically eliminate the desire to share bad information about anyone else.

For the Trainer

After reading chapter 11, either on your own or as a group, discuss the following:

1. How do you handle gossip? What would you say or do if a colleague approached you to talk poorly about someone else?
2. Have you ever been harmed by gossip? If so, how did you handle it?

12

Mindful Communications

Your time is limited so don't waste it living someone else's life.

—STEVE JOBS

The damaging power of negative speech is exceeded only by the constructive power of positive speech. Admiring and speaking encouragingly about others benefits not only ourselves but the people being praised as well. The Venerable Wonji Dharma, a brilliant Buddhist priest and scholar, taught me a simple yet helpful communication tool. "Before speaking," he said, "THINK: is what I'm about to say **T**rue, **H**elpful, **I**nspiring, **N**ecessary, and **K**ind? If not, don't say it."

Thoughts and Words

Mindful communications involve becoming aware of our thinking and the choices we make in communicating. Like any mindfulness, it is about being fully present in the moment. When we are mindful of our communications, we are conscious of the words we are choosing. We are therefore less likely to regret how we speak in a challenging situation. We are also less likely to take things personally when we communicate with full presence. If you tend to already be thinking about what you are going to say while the other person is still talking, you are not being fully present, which diminishes your ability to truly listen. Be genuine and learn to listen without judgment to what the other person wants to convey.

If we want to create a positive work culture, we must base our practices on respect and caring. To honor our ethics and values as an organization, we have to begin by respecting each other's humanity so we can connect as fully as possible. I have always taught mindful communication to my graduate-level business communication classes with this very goal in mind.

Being Fully Present

Another important part of mindful communication is becoming comfortable with silence. Allow the people you are speaking with to collect their thoughts or feel the feelings coming up for them at that moment. Don't rush them or try to lead the conversation. Give them the time they need to express themselves fully, and you will find your conversation far more meaningful. A common complaint I often hear from veterinary professionals is that the "administration doesn't care." Many have said that if they are given a chance to speak with an administrator about a problem or complaint, they are rushed through it and typically told why they are wrong to feel the way they do. Some administrators take control of the conversation immediately, talk very quickly, give little time to respond, tell them why they are wrong, and then excuse them. Not one of these professionals has come away from the conversation feeling heard; most say that it was a complete waste of their time and see it as evidence that their thoughts and feelings don't matter.

For managers and administrators, it doesn't matter how intelligent you are, how many great concepts you have offered, or how many talented people you have hired. What matters is that you communicate with your teams so that they walk away from your discussions feeling heard and valued. Find the courage to open up your heart and let your guard down. Open yourself fully to whomever you are speaking to while being respectfully attuned to the timing and the space you are in. By being authentic, you will help others do the same. Be mindful of not entering the communication with an agenda. Take only your curiosity and the desire to understand into the room. Instead of consecutive monologues, mindful communication will allow you to fully experience what the other person is trying to share with you and give you greater awareness.

Communication is a form of piloting between at least two living beings, each with their own ways of looking at things as well as their own histories, ideas, and beliefs. With mindful communication, we can change how we communicate to focus not only on listening and speaking but also on an inner aspect: consciousness. Showing up for a conversation or meeting and ensuring we have fully arrived before speaking is an essential first step. The most valuable conversations will result from joining together our mindful objectives with our mindful actions.

We must give our full attention to whomever we are speaking to, moment by moment. Suppose we are thinking about something other than what we are talking about. In that case, the probability of us missing the mark and not understanding fully is high, and our communication partner will most often perceive it. Remember, our goal in conversation is to gain further understanding, not to prove ourselves or show why we are correct. The connection we create can then become the basis for meaningful and helpful discussions with members of the veterinary team or the other animal-care professionals with whom we work.

For the Trainer

After reading chapter 12, either on your own or as a group, discuss the following:

1. Are you comfortable with silence when in the presence of others? Why or why not?
2. What can you do to make your verbal communications more effective?

13

Introvert and Extrovert Personality Types

Change your thoughts and you change your world.

—NORMAN VINCENT PEALE

As you have seen, just because you are compassionate toward others does not mean you are compassionate toward yourself or your own suffering. In fact, it is not uncommon to see kind and compassionate veterinary or other animal-care professionals who leave themselves no room for imperfection. This explains, at least in part, why veterinary medicine still has such high numbers of suicides every year.

The Myers-Briggs Type Indicator (MBTI), referred to in chapter 3, indicates that perfectionists overshadow the field of veterinary medicine. Sadly, a significant correlation exists in the general population between perfectionistic personalities and, according to a study published in the Journal of Personality, suicidal ideation and suicide attempts (Smith et al. 2018). Tragically, there is also a high correlation between introverted adolescents and suicide. Additionally, the MBTI indicates that a large percentage of those attracted to a life in veterinary medicine are introverts (Goetz et al. 2020). This fact, coupled with the emotionally taxing and all too often traumatic work that veterinary and animal-care professionals face daily, along with the potential for cyberbullying and gossip, makes it easy to understand why those devastating numbers have tragically remained high.

Personality Traits of Introverts

Introverts are more focused on internal thoughts and feelings than external ones. According to many personality theorists, everyone has some degree of both introversion and extroversion. Most people fall somewhere between the two, although some tend to lean toward one more than the other. Dr. Dan McAdams, chair of the Psychology Department at Northwestern University, described extroversion and introversion as a "continuous dimension," meaning that there are no pure types. He indicated that, as with any continuous scale, there will always be people who score in the extremes, but most will fall somewhere in the middle. Approximately one-quarter of our population identifies with introversion. The introversion-extroversion measurement is also one of the four areas the MBTI identifies.

Introverts tend to enjoy thinking deeply about things and researching topics of interest. They also tend to be very self-aware and therefore understand themselves more than others typically might. Because introverts believe understanding themselves is important, they will often devote time to learning more about themselves. This might involve exploring meditation, yoga, and their ancestries; learning about religions, cultures, philosophy, psychology, biology, astrology, and numerology; or researching other themes they find interesting. If you tend to be self-aware and appreciate gathering knowledge about yourself, introversion might be part of your personality profile.

According to Dr. Hans Eysenck's book *Dimensions of Personality*, introverts have high arousal levels. Therefore, Eysenck says introverts tend to have a higher comfort level with events, people, and places without too much stimulation. They are more alert than nonintroverts and more affected by their environments. Finding a place to be alone to recharge tends to be necessary for most introverts (Eysenck 1997).

On a physiological level, the neurons in the reticular activating system (RAS) in our brains regulate the amount of stimulation we experience. The RAS also plays a role in determining the amount of information we absorb. Arousal levels are increased by the RAS when we find ourselves confronted by possible threats. It increases our levels of stimulation in such situations to alert us to potential threats.

The common signs of an introvert include becoming emotionally exhausted by being around a large number of people; preferring to be in the company of a small gathering of close friends as opposed to large parties; appreciating alone time, especially when surrounded by people all day; tending to have a smaller group of close friends; preferring one-on-one conversations and interactions as opposed to large group venues; appearing quiet or reserved; being overwhelmed by hectic environments; tending to be self-aware; learning most effectively by observation; enjoying working independently; and preferring to practice tasks in private.

An assumption many people make is that introverts are shy, which is incorrect. Shyness has more to do with the stress or discomfort of being around other people. Because introverts tend to think before they talk, they do not typically enjoy idle conversation; they are more inclined to enjoy deep and meaningful discussions.

I have always been regarded as an introvert. Being alone helps me recharge, as it does for most introverts. But our society taught me to develop my ability to act the opposite to "fit in" and be taken seriously. I much prefer to be alone or to share a meaningful conversation or positive experience with one to three good friends. I have never enjoyed anything loud, including large parties, loud voices, lawnmowers, booming music, and so on. At my seventh birthday party, after only one hour, I asked my mother to please send all my guests home. She was surprised and asked me why. "They are so loud and so wild," I told her. I have always preferred calm environments.

Differences Between Introverts and Extroverts

Introversion and extroversion appear to exist at opposite ends of the same scale. Introverts typically focus on their own thoughts and feelings rather than anything or anyone outside themselves. Introverts tend to be hypersensitive and need to isolate themselves to revitalize, especially after having been around a lot of people. Extroverts, on the other hand, seem to be energized through socialization. Ambiverts are those who, at times, enjoy being alone and, at other times, like being in the company of others.

Response to Environment and Communication Styles

Like everything else, our physical reactions to our surroundings are not always a choice. They indicate how we experience and respond to various aspects of our environment. It is a completely individual experience and plays a formative role in defining our tendencies toward either introversion or extroversion. Neither category is bad or good, and neither is right or wrong; it just is.

Because of the amount of speaking I do, many people assume I am an extrovert. It's a common mistake: introverts may be outwardly very social and enjoy large gatherings. Not all introverts prefer to be at home with a good book while surrounded by their cherished pets. I, like many introverts, have higher arousal levels, so I have always sought out solitude or, at a minimum, nonchaotic environments. For instance, when speaking at a veterinary conference, I will not sign up for any of the conference meals and will always disappear just before the big conference party begins. They are so loud, and so much is going on that none of my colleagues have ever caught my disappearing act. In fact, over the years, many have asked whether I enjoyed myself at the party! If I am overwhelmed by being around a lot of people while working, I will commonly go to my car and simply observe my breath for five or ten minutes. If I don't have five or ten minutes, I will take refuge in the restroom for a couple of minutes and, believe it or not, it helps. You might be surprised to learn who in your work or social circle is or is not an introvert. Some introverts present themselves very differently than they feel and can be very social.

Introverts tend to take in more information from their environments. Escaping somewhere to have time alone to recharge gives them the opportunity to regroup, but some introverts actually enjoy socializing (Eysenck 1997). As an introvert, I enjoy being alone. As a mother of several children and someone with a practice that involves giving my attention to clients daily, that may sound very odd. Don't get me wrong, I have always enjoyed every second I have with my loved ones and still find my work extremely fulfilling. However, I do need my alone time. It doesn't have to be for a long period; an hour or two can feel like a vacation and be highly rejuvenating. Although I don't love huge social gatherings, I adore coming together with my closest friends, colleagues, and mentors with whom I can share real conversations.

It's extremely useful to be aware of the variance in how different personality types communicate to help us more fully comprehend ourselves and the people with whom we interact. Veterinary and animal-care professionals spend long hours under stressful conditions with each other, so it is essential to understand that we all have different ways of doing things. The most important thing is to respect and honor those differences between ourselves and others.

The differences between introverts and extroverts can be attributed to our physical makeup and consequential bodily responses to our environments. As one example, extroverts tend to be energized by social interactions, whereas, as we have examined, introverts tend to be exhausted or easily overwhelmed by being around too many people. Extroverts therefore may mistakenly think of introverts as being shy or unfriendly because they don't understand how introverts typically operate. They often cannot understand why someone would want to be alone.

There are far more extroverts than introverts in our population, approximately three to one. Several introverts have told me they are tired of their colleagues or friends trying to change them to become more social. But don't forget, approximately 70 percent identify with characteristics of both introversion and extroversion. Ambiverts can easily enjoy aspects of both (Davidson 2017).

It appears to be extremely difficult for extroverts to understand how introverts operate. One of my daughters is an extrovert and cannot understand why anyone would prefer to be alone "doing nothing." She still struggles with the idea and thinks nobody would truly want to be alone if given a choice. No matter how often I have tried to explain the issue to extroverts, I have never sensed that any of them truly understood, including my daughter! One thing you can keep in mind is that no matter what type you are, one type isn't superior to the other. Each has its unique attributes.

Introverts tend to do better when they have a strong social support network and when they are aware of a few useful emotional regulation skills. It is not uncommon for introverts to struggle with anxiety. Life can sometimes feel overwhelming when we feel our thoughts and emotions so deeply. Mindfulness-based living can provide an effective way of dealing with anxiety, as can meditation, journaling, exercising, and walks in nature. If you still struggle, I suggest contacting a mental health professional and seeking the help you deserve.

Nothing is more valuable than knowing ourselves well and understanding how we tend to operate as individuals. Perhaps the suicide rates in veterinary medicine could finally subside if we learned how to honor and respect our differences and worked with them to take good care of ourselves and others.

I highly suggest taking the Myers-Briggs Type Indicator if you haven't done so already. Learning how you take in information, why certain things are of interest to you, and why you react to certain situations or certain people the way you do has the potential to help you better understand yourself. It can also give you the ability to understand why others operate the way they do, thus increasing your ability to be more compassionate toward yourself and others. The MBTI can be found at www.myersbriggs.org.

For the Trainer

After reading chapter 13, either on your own or as a group, discuss the following:

1. Do you consider yourself an introvert, extrovert, or ambivert? Why?
2. If you have taken the Myers-Briggs Type Indicator, what personality type are you?
3. Do you find it useful to know these things about yourself? If so, why?
4. Do you think that this information will help you understand others?

14

The Tragedy of Suicide

As you grow older, you will discover that you have two hands; one for helping yourself, and the other for helping others.

—AUDREY HEPBURN

Tragically, Dr. Shirley Koshi, Dr. Sophia Yin, Dr. Tiffany Margolin, and Dr. Amanda Lumsden are not the only veterinarians I've known who have used suicide as an escape from the enormity of their pain since the first edition of this book was released in 2013. My goal at that time was to get the word out on compassion fatigue to stop so many veterinary and animal-care professionals from considering suicide a viable option, which it's still not. Because a number of veterinary university programs are using the book as mandatory reading and because one such university designed a class around the book, I had a false sense of comfort that my goal was being reached and that the word was indeed getting out to veterinary communities. With the current statistics of one in six veterinarians in the US having contemplated suicide, I now know that getting the word out was only the beginning, and sadly, it's just not enough (Tomasi et al. 2019).

Together, we must bring down our devastating suicide numbers. First and foremost, we must begin by changing our cultural view of asking for help. Please help me alleviate the stigma around mental health issues. Let's create a culture based on kindness, where people are honored for having the courage to speak up and ask for the help they need and deserve. We are all the same,

Important Resources

If you suspect a colleague may be contemplating suicide, never hesitate to contact the National Suicide Prevention Lifeline—even if you are not sure. It's better to be wrong than not to have tried: call 1-800-273-8255 or SMS text 988.

I am grateful that the number of veterinary organizations offering suicide-prevention support, in general, is increasing, and I would like to thank the following compassionate groups and associations:

- The American Animal Hospital Association (AAHA), for being there from the beginning and increasing awareness about compassion fatigue through the books they publish and the continuing education they offer. Additionally, the AAHA has set the uppermost standards in their associated companion-animal veterinary hospitals to provide the highest possible care to pets, their families, and the veterinary teams.
- The American Veterinary Medical Association (AVMA), for offering a free online training course that helps veterinarians identify suicidal ideation in others and know how to refer colleagues they fear may be at risk. They also provide an article, "Updates from the AVMA Feature Resource to Combat Cyberbullying," which everyone in the veterinary and animal-care professions should read (Nolen 2023a).
- Not One More Vet (NOMV 2023), for the thousands of veterinarians who find support and comfort every day through their online private support group for veterinarians.
- Banfield Hospitals, for their recent generous offering of online suicide-prevention classes, which are complimentary to all those in the veterinary field.
- The American Foundation for Suicide Prevention (afsp.org), for providing mental health support and suicide prevention resources, on a complimentary basis, for those going through a particularly difficult time.

and we all have the same feelings; therefore, there is no feeling we should be ashamed of. If you have felt it, so have I. Feelings don't define us; they simply make us human and are something we all share. Feelings are fleeting. All that defines us is how we treat others and ourselves, moment by moment. Stop holding yourself to standards you don't expect from anyone else. Shine the light of your compassion that you give so readily to everyone else on yourself, and let's see if we can't turn the suicide numbers around.

Everyone should be aware of and able to recognize the warning signs of suicide, whether for themselves or someone else. Education on suicide, and the most effective way to intervene, should be a part of every veterinary or animal-care professional's job training.

Every one of us can help prevent suicide. The most common warning signs of someone contemplating or planning suicide are many and varied. Some are subtle, and others are more clear indications that someone is in danger and may urgently need help:

- Increase in drug or alcohol use
- Talking about being a burden; feeling empty
- Feeling like they have no way out of their problems
- Feeling guilty or ashamed
- Talking about having no reason to live
- Saying that others would be better off without them
- Talking about seeking revenge or beginning to exhibit rage
- Withdrawing and/or isolating
- Sleeping significantly more or less
- Displaying extreme mood swings
- Giving away their personal possessions
- Suddenly starting to tie up loose ends
- Feeling hopeless
- Acting uncharacteristically anxious, agitated, or reckless
- Talking about wanting to die or about dying in general
- Suffering from untreated depression
- Accessing lethal means, such as stockpiling pills
- Changes in personality, such as a gentle person becoming aggressive

For the Trainer

After reading chapter 14, either on your own or as a group, discuss the following:

1. In general, are you comfortable asking for help? Why or why not?
2. Do you hold yourself to higher standards than you do anyone else? If so, why do you think that is?

15

Resilience

If your compassion does not include yourself, it is incomplete.

—JACK KORNFIELD

***Resilience* is the reliance on our own strengths and resources to see us through life** or hard times, as opposed to continually relying on others. Resilient people believe in themselves and don't allow adversity to dissuade them. They acknowledge that bad times may happen, but that doesn't define them. Rather, they view bad times as a difficult yet temporary phase through which they must pass. Self-resiliency is illustrated by the ability to prepare yourself, mentally and emotionally, to stay mindful and present to whatever life brings while knowing that, because of your sense of purpose, you will meet all the challenges just as you will meet all the joy.

Characteristics of Resilient People

Resilient people tend to be self-aware and therefore more conscious of the feelings and cues of those around them. They tend to know when it's time to leave or dive in and when it's time to ask for help or offer it. If guitar strings are wound too tightly, they will break when hit by something, whereas if those same strings are more flexible, they will make music instead of breaking. Just like the strings of a guitar, people can be fragile and susceptible to damage when subjected to excessive tension. In contrast, those who maintain a sense of calm in good or bad times can help themselves and those around them. Resilient people support others well and lend a sense of calm through their encouragement.

Self-resilient people practice tolerance, knowing that "this too shall pass," an idea that applies to nearly every bad situation. Resilient people also understand that pain and suffering are a part of living; that such things come and go from our lives. As hard as it is in the moment, it's more beneficial to come to terms with the truth of pain than to ignore, repress, or deny it. Acceptance is about leaning into the negative experience and learning from it while knowing that, eventually, we will be okay. Being present to what is by staying mindful of what we are experiencing, without judging it or trying to run from it, will strengthen our resilience and allow us to recuperate rapidly to normal functioning after facing adversity. Many veterinary and animal-care professionals adapt to challenges by pulling from their natural strengths. However, because of the ongoing intensity and number of distressing situations they commonly attend to, most of these professionals will need to build their resilience intentionally. This is essential to counterbalance the effects of long-term exposure to mental, physical, and emotional stress.

Creating a Veterinary Resilience Plan

Whether you are part of a veterinary team, an animal rescuer, or an animal shelter worker, you would be well advised to develop a plan to become more resilient to the ongoing challenges you face in your profession. Whether from continual emergencies or ongoing chronic stress, these challenges have the potential to significantly affect your overall well-being. Those who are struggling with this kind of ongoing stress tend to suffer more severe consequences when their support networks are unavailable. In such situations, you will typically need more time to recover. Building our resilience generally reduces the impact on our health, careers, relationships, and the amount of time it takes us to recover from traumatic situations. So, focusing on ways to decrease vulnerability and increase resilience can benefit the entire animal-care community by improving overall health and well-being.

Creating resilience may require reframing current approaches to well-being in veterinary practice. Social connections affect resilience, which can affect our capacity to continue in difficult and often traumatic work. As a result, social systems are often formed between veterinary and animal-care professionals. Working environments that encourage social connectedness show higher rates of resilience, which then serves veterinary professionals well when dealing with particularly difficult cases. Strong ties can more efficiently mobilize and connect team members so they can help each other overcome painful or difficult situations. Resilience training can improve the efficiency of recovering from particularly painful cases.

We all face painful and tragic moments in our lives; no one is immune. As noted earlier, suffering is a part of life. However, we have the choice to allow adversity to teach us and help us grow and realize our strengths, or to let it destroy us. There are things that boost our resilience. Working with grieving clients for the past twenty years and having dealt with my own losses, I know well that we all need a sense of hope when dealing with the loss of a beloved one. We can find that hope and rise above our pain through our thoughts and actions toward others.

Coping with Trauma and Loss

Resilient people tend not to personalize the trauma and losses they face. Instead of feeling that they are being punished or unfairly treated, they accept that difficult things are a part of life. Some events or circumstances cannot be changed no matter what we do. What matters is that we carefully choose how to think when something horrible happens. Being able to shift the focus of your attention to something positive can be very influential. There can be happy thoughts even with the pain; one does not exclude the other.

Change is a constant, and resilience allows us to ride the waves of change while adapting to the new normal and recovering as soon as possible. We can learn from our mistakes and rebound from our failures. With a positive attitude and perspective, we can overcome anything. I'm not saying it will be easy, but you can do it. Let tragedy teach you so you can become more compassionate and help others. Resilient people tend to be healthier and happier than those who are not and, as a result, tend to recover faster from pain. Be kind to yourself and others—we are all in this together. To help cultivate this, consider this exercise. Before starting work each day, breathe thoughtfully in and out a few times and then ask yourself what your intention is for the day. After work, ask yourself what you can let go of from that day and then give yourself permission to do just that.

From a different perspective, veterinary and animal-care professionals enter the field partly because of their nature and values, which may arise from their sense of spirituality. While they may represent many different faith perspectives, they find themselves dealing with similar questions in response to suffering and injustice. Additionally, research shows that those with a deep sense of spirituality are more resilient in the face of trauma (VHA 2020). A sense of connectedness can originate from organized religion, but feeling deeply connected can also be the product of a strong sense of relationship to nature—to animals, the earth, the ocean, or trees. Bring whatever gives you that sense of connectedness into your life regularly to help expand your resilience.

For the Trainer

After reading chapter 15, either on your own or as a group, discuss the following:

1. Do you consider yourself a resilient person? Why or why not?
2. What gives you a deep sense of connectedness?

PART IV

TREATING COMPASSION FATIGUE

16

No Script, No Road Map

All the darkness of the world cannot extinguish the light of a small candle.

—SAINT FRANCIS OF ASSISI

Although we know that both internal and external factors are at work in compassion fatigue, we also understand that these combine uniquely for every individual. The immediate causes are unique to every individual, and every individual has a different set of strengths and weaknesses, coping mechanisms, and so on. For all these reasons, it's important to understand that there is no script or road map for dealing with the effects of compassion fatigue.

The emotional climate of your work setting plays a role, as does the level of support you are offered. Your personality, temperament, level of connection, personal support system, personal history, and the intensity of your losses all play a role in determining the intensity of your response.

In some ways, it would be much easier if there were simple, black-and-white rules to follow. But dealing with continual trauma and grief isn't easy work. There are no precedents on which you can rely because no one else is exactly like you. Being a caregiver can be a bit like bodysurfing: sometimes we find ourselves riding the waves with ease, when suddenly a huge, unexpected wave rises behind us and takes us out, making us crash violently to the depths of the ocean floor. Working effectively with grief and trauma—ours or someone else's—requires us to know how to ride these waves. Again, it's about balance, but everyone has a different way of finding that balance. Some people do best by verbally expressing their pain, whereas others benefit from doing something physical (and we discuss both methods in later chapters).

Having easy, black-and-white rules would mean that all the waves were the same and all the surfers were the same. And what surfer would ever want that? Life is a challenge, and because of our unique challenges, we can grow and become wave dancers.

Determining Your Emotional Triggers

Almost everyone has certain triggers that cause them to recall their own losses and traumas from the past. A trigger is a stimulus that brings about an emotional response. It can be elicited by any one of the five senses. In other words, something you see, hear, touch, smell, or taste can take you right back to a painful and traumatic loss or experience, and for a moment, you may find yourself experiencing it all over again.

For one veterinary technician, it was the smell of jasmine. Whenever jasmine was in bloom, she would remember sitting in her yard with her beloved pug as they played, relaxed, or just spent time together. This smell triggered a painful and sad response. For another veterinary caregiver, the smell of turkey cooking in the oven triggered memories. In her case, the memories were of her father, who had died on Thanksgiving. She had been very close to him; every Thanksgiving, she again grieves his death. These individuals couldn't avoid the smell of jasmine or Thanksgiving turkey. But by knowing their triggers, they could prepare themselves and deal with the memories proactively, thus reducing their potential impact on their lives.

Triggers can also be specific dates, days of the week, or times of the day. These are calendar triggers. One veterinarian I knew became visibly depressed and hypersensitive every Tuesday after the traumatic loss of her dog, who had died on a Tuesday afternoon. Another struggled on the twenty-third of every month, the day she lost her beloved cat. Surprisingly, calendar triggers can occur whether or not the person is consciously aware of the date and time.

The important thing is to become aware of our individual triggers so we can be as prepared as possible for what will likely follow. This is easier to do when the triggers are predictable, recurring events, such as something that occurs in a specific season (the blooming of jasmine), on a given holiday (the smell of turkey), or on a given day (calendar triggers). I suggest keeping a grief journal and including a section for triggers. When something causes a painful emotional response or remembrance of your loss, write it down in your trigger section. In this way, you can begin to track what your triggers are so you can be prepared for them.

What we cannot predict or prepare for are unexpected triggers. We cannot predict our reactions when listening to accounts of the traumatic experiences of others, such as clients, or when we are involved in helping them through the traumatic experience itself. This is why we must be prepared for whatever wave may come. To do that, we must follow a proactive regimen to support ourselves. If we do, we will not be tempted to turn toward self-destructive behaviors, such as acting without regard for the consequences of our actions or attempting to numb ourselves to the pain.

Just as the intensity of a relationship dictates the intensity of the grieving process, there is a correlation between traumatic material and the negative effects that exposure to it may have. As we know, exposure to life-and-death situations is high in the work of veterinary professionals. It can be traumatizing,

Case Study | Janet

"I can't do this anymore," said Janet, a highly regarded veterinary oncology technician at a specialty clinic, one dark and enormously sad morning. She had been dealing with a number of stressors: client expectations, anxiety in the practice's atmosphere, lack of personal time, and physical and mental exhaustion. At that point, she hit a horrible bump in the road that sent her straight into the arms of compassion fatigue and a temporary state of paralysis. An adorable two-year-old West Highland terrier she had been treating for cancer accidentally fell into the family pool and died.

To make matters worse, the entire department had celebrated the terrier's recovery less than a month previously. The owners had brought her in for one last recheck, and she had been deemed a graduate of her cancer treatment. Everyone felt very close to both the clients and the patient, who had been coming to the practice two to four times every week. Shock and sorrow riveted the department when the phone call came in and the grieving owners reported that the little Westie had drowned.

The technician—who had fallen in love with this sweet dog and her family—was devastated, and the veterinary field lost another wonderful professional. However, there is a chance that if Janet had been using self-care strategies all along, she would not have reacted this way. She was already vulnerable to losing her balance when the call came in.

continually exposing caregivers to the risk of compassion fatigue (see textbox "Case Study: Janet").

Learning to take care of yourself will not happen all at once, especially if you are not accustomed to making self-care a priority. It will take practice. The important thing is to begin somewhere. By beginning self-care strategies, you will immediately notice incremental improvement.

Taking the First Steps

The only way through the pain and confusion of compassion fatigue is by recognizing, honoring, and expressing your pain while remaining proactive in your self-care. As a veterinary professional, you must have a place where you feel safe to express your emotions as they come up. It may not be easy, but it is imperative that you do this to find your sense of balance again.

Later chapters offer specific suggestions about how to be proactive in your battle against compassion fatigue. But you can take a small step in the right direction today. You probably already know some things that work for you—it's just that you never actually do them. If you feel better after taking a walk in the park, by all means, go out and do it. If you benefit from putting on your headphones and listening to classical music in your comfy chair, going to the gym and working out, or having lunch with your best friend—then do those things. Maybe a good night's sleep and a day of rest always helps you feel relaxed. The important thing is to get started.

Although you can take your first steps today, remember that the journey to recovery may be long. You will need to learn how to express and process your emotions, which may take some time. Repairing damaged relationships also takes time. As you begin to use the self-care strategies you already know, continue to read this book to learn new ones.

Do not expect the journey to recovery to be easy. Certain life experiences can predispose caregivers to more severe and even pathological responses to grief and compassion fatigue. It is important to follow up further in such cases; this process also takes time. An expert in the field of compassion fatigue can help. If you have a limited social support system, live alone, have recently suffered a significant loss, find yourself thinking about death and suicide, or have a history of mental illness or depression, it is imperative to seek out the additional support you both need and deserve. In this case, your first step may be making a phone call to your doctor to ask about a referral.

As you begin to take care of yourself, you will start to notice that your burden seems to be lightening, bit by bit. You will be better positioned to ride any unexpected waves that might come along because you will begin to regain your balance. Stick with it; your journey has just begun.

For the Trainer

After reading chapter 16, meet as a group and complete this exercise together.

1. This chapter discusses emotional triggers, events, and sensory experiences that cause you to recall earlier times in your life. Sometimes these are negative memories, such as the memory of a trauma. Sometimes they are positive memories. Can you identify such triggers in your life? Bring notebooks or hand out paper and pens and give group members fifteen minutes to journal privately about this question. As you come together as a group after the journaling exercise, ask group members, on a voluntary basis, to share some of their thoughts about triggers and how they have played a role in their lives.
2. Then, allow another ten minutes or so for group members to do the following exercise: This chapter discusses taking the first steps toward preventing or recovering from compassion fatigue. Brainstorm on your own to jot down ideas for self-care strategies that you already know work well for you. As a group, share some of these ideas. Notice that there may be a wide range of self-care strategies mentioned because everyone is different. This week, your mission is to implement one of the ideas you know works for you. If someone else has an idea that you have never tried, experiment with that idea as well.

Note to group leader: for the next session, there is a guest speaker suggestion in the "For the Trainer" section. If you would like to use this suggestion, be sure to arrange for this before the next group session.

17

Getting Help

Finding a Compassion Fatigue Specialist

Don't ask yourself what the world needs; ask yourself what makes you come alive. And then go and do that. Because what the world needs is people who have come alive.

—HOWARD THURMAN

It is easy for veterinary professionals to become consumed by the exhaustion and despair that accompanies endless and ongoing human and animal suffering. No matter your dreams or how much energy you started with in your profession, reality can insidiously erode it all if you do not take care to prevent compassion fatigue.

Your love for animals was an incredible motivation to enter the profession; however, it can backfire on you if you don't get a handle on your emotional responses to the trauma you encounter routinely. If you don't learn to process these emotions, the work you once loved can eventually cause you great harm. You may find yourself unable to continue in the field—your personal and family life could become a wreck, or your health might be ruined. It's that important. If you neglect your needs by always putting your work first and never taking the time to nurture yourself, you will more than likely fall victim to compassion fatigue. You are a compassionate human being, not an invincible superhuman made of steel. Compassionate human beings will experience negative repercussions if they try to hold all those feelings inside.

The good news is that you can thrive again once you learn to process your emotions in a positive way. This involves being compassionate and nonjudgmental toward yourself. That same kindness and understanding you offer to others without question is something you should give to yourself. When others fail, you are understanding toward them, and you should also be understanding toward yourself. The first step in expressing your emotions and releasing them is accepting them. They are what they are. Know that you are having these emotions because you are a compassionate person. You never treat others harshly when they are suffering, nor should you treat yourself harshly.

As caregivers, we are adept at absorbing the trauma and suffering of others, and we must learn to release the painful feelings we accumulate. However, we cannot just dump all these emotions on whomever is close by. We cannot share too many traumatic experiences with our family and friends because we would leave them with potentially toxic images. It is better to seek out a caregiving support group, a compassion fatigue specialist, or a mental health professional familiar with pet loss or compassion fatigue. Also, doing something physical or creative can be a helpful outlet. Take care of yourself physically, mentally, emotionally, and spiritually, but do not burden your loved ones with the baggage you are trying to shed. That approach will only leave them exhausted as well. In this chapter, we look at how to find a professional who can help you process your emotions. Chapter 18 looks at other healthy ways to let go of these burdensome feelings.

Finding a Compassion Fatigue Specialist

Someone who listens to those who are traumatized, afraid, grieving, or suffering from compassion fatigue must, above all, want to listen and understand. It was to fill this need that the field of veterinary support and pet-loss recovery was born. One reason this is a specialized field of expertise is that not all specialists understand the intense and complex emotions surrounding pet loss and veterinary caregiving. Finding someone who understands veterinary issues and will not try to minimize the pain is essential. It can be counterproductive if you attempt to "make do" with a professional who is not right for the job. In the following, I share some of my personal experiences in the hope that it will help you find someone who can truly help you recover from compassion fatigue or prevent it from occurring.

How (Not) to Find a Good Listener

To take care of yourself, you will need to express your feelings, which means you will need to find someone who can listen. I learned the hard way that it is sometimes difficult to find the right counselor. More than fifteen years ago, my precious three-year-old yellow Lab Cheyenne's cancer diagnosis became a life-altering experience for me. I knew I needed to find someone to talk to. Not knowing any better at that time, I sought help from a former colleague in the Beverly Hills area who is a clinical psychologist. She had always seemed competent, knowledgeable, and kind, so I called her office and booked an appointment.

I knew that what I felt after Cheyenne's terminal diagnosis was anticipatory grief. Anticipatory grief typically begins the moment a terminal diagnosis is made, and it can painfully bring up the same dreadful emotions associated with the loss of a loved one. I was looking forward to finally having someone to talk to who could help me through my difficult feelings. But my hopes were soon crushed. I sat in the chair opposite the psychologist and told her what had brought me in. Her face was shocked and confused as she responded, "Wait a minute, you are here because you are grieving for a dog?" I couldn't speak. I just looked at her, got up, placed my check on her desk, and walked out. Although this very intelligent woman holds a doctorate in clinical psychology, she was not familiar with the intensity of pet-loss issues, nor could she relate to my loss on a personal level. She was clearly not someone I should have been talking to about my grief.

What a disappointment. As I drove home that day, all I could think was, "Now what do I do with all of this fear and sadness that is welling up inside me?" I had my animals, my practice, and a family to look after, and I was having trouble concentrating and staying on task. It was a disaster! I then began my search for someone who would understand, beginning with my immediate area and then expanding outward. I was willing to go just about anywhere, but I could find no one who specialized in pet-loss support.

Finally, I came across the name of a woman who had a practice about three hours from my home. She had a pet-loss support group closer to my home once a month. The group met about halfway between her practice and where I lived. After searching for so long, I thought an hour-and-a-half car ride seemed completely reasonable, and I felt fortunate.

The day finally came for the group's next gathering, and I drove the distance, making a special effort to get there early so I could find parking. I didn't want to be late and miss a moment of the two-hour meeting. I carefully chose my seat in the circle of chairs before me. The group facilitator was at her desk and did not acknowledge me. Slowly, people started coming in, and the circle was quickly filled. The facilitator joined the group, sitting in the seat facing the front door that she had saved for herself. She started the group by inviting people to talk about their grief and how they were faring.

But to my shock and dismay, the woman I had so looked forward to meeting was so visibly uninterested in what was being shared that she looked more at her watch than she did at the faces of pain before her. It seemed as if the people who had been there before knew the drill; they told their stories in an almost robotic fashion, whereas the newer ones were so swallowed up by their tears that they could barely speak. This woman never responded to their upwelling of emotion. Her expression rarely changed, her empathetic response was nonexistent, and truly, the only things she showed any interest in whatsoever were her watch and the checks we wrote out to her at the end of the session.

I felt so unsafe and so much more vulnerable after witnessing her behavior that I chose to pass when it came to telling my story. To make matters worse, at the end of the group, while the facilitator collected her fees, one distraught individual, who appeared to be genuinely embarrassed, said, "I am so sorry, I forgot to grab my checkbook. May I give it to you next time?" to which our supposed healer replied, "Do you mind getting paid a month after you do your work? Payment is due at the time services are rendered. I thought that I was clear about that." Feeling horrible for him yet equally as powerless, I couldn't wait to slam yet another check down as I raced to my car. I was overwhelmed by my disappointment and feelings of helplessness.

Once my shock began to subside, I slowly found myself becoming embarrassed that a fellow professional would take advantage of such a vulnerable population as those who were grieving. My disappointment turned to anger. Now what? The anger was a great place to hide for a while, but that lasted only a moment in the grand scheme of things.

I knew what had to be done, and I knew I had to do it. I approached the owner of the specialty practice that was treating my Cheyenne, and he readily agreed to allow me to volunteer my services and run a pet-loss support group once a month out of his facility. Not knowing how to market it, I relied on word of mouth, and to my surprise, our group grew quickly. Many people drove long distances, just as I had, to find someone who understood. Soon our monthly group met twice a month, and not long after that, we began to come together weekly. The numbers just kept growing.

During the nine years I ran the pet-loss support group at that specialty practice, our group grew so much that we could no longer fit into the treatment room designated for us. At that time in my life, I decided to devote my entire professional career to veterinary support and pet-loss recovery. I already held a doctorate in clinical psychology and returned to school to earn certification in grief recovery. That's when one of the most rewarding chapters in my life began.

Let my experiences from fifteen years ago serve as a lesson to you. Do not go to just any professional. If you go to the first session and realize that the specialist is not the right one for you, pay for that appointment but do not make another one. To have better success than I did, follow the guidelines in the next section.

How to Find a Good Listener

Fortunately, the specialty involving veterinary issues has become much better understood today than it was fifteen years ago. With any luck, you will not have such a hard time finding a specialist who understands pet loss, trauma, and compassion fatigue that you have to go back to school to become certified yourself! As a veterinary practice employee, you probably already know some professionals dealing with veterinary issues. Start there.

When seeking someone to help with compassion fatigue, remember that educational background does not always indicate effectiveness in this line of work. To provide successful support for veterinary caregivers, specialists must have felt the depth of the love and intensity that can exist in the relationships we share with pets. If they have felt this bond, they will be able to understand the trauma your clients encounter when they are threatened with the loss of that love. They will also understand why the secondary trauma you are experiencing is so overwhelming. Just as important, they must want to listen, not for a paycheck or because they feel they have to, but because they truly want to be there without judgment or the need to fix anything.

Appropriate specialists will have experience with the issues surrounding veterinary caregiving and compassion fatigue. They should be able to remain nonjudgmental and be compassionate and kind. In a session with them, you should not feel as if you have to do anything more than be there at that moment and be fully present. You should feel safe and accepted when in a session.

If you do not already know of good specialists in your area who work with pet-loss recovery and other veterinary mental-health issues, then you will need to find them. You need to compile that list anyway to have somewhere to send clients who are struggling with grief. Ask other veterinarians in your area for recommendations. You can also go to pet-loss websites to find a list of licensed professionals in your area who work with veterinary issues, or you can google keywords such as "veterinary compassion fatigue" and the name of your city and state.

Don't feel that you have to already be on the brink of breaking down completely before seeking help. A good compassion fatigue specialist can teach you preventive strategies so that you will be equipped to deal with the traumas that confront you. It's good preventive medicine. Being proactive in our stance against compassion fatigue is the only way to ensure that we will not become victims of it.

It's important to maintain a place where you can go to debrief regularly. Once you find your compassion fatigue specialist, keep up that relationship. Once you find your balance, you may not have to meet every week or every month, but do keep up the dialogue at a level that seems right for you. In that way, you can prevent compassion fatigue from recurring.

For the Trainer

Note that item 3 below includes a guest speaker suggestion. The group leader may opt to arrange for this in advance. Also, the group leader should bring to this session a list of specialists in the local area who deal with compassion fatigue and/or pet loss, with a copy for each member of the group. If desired, include a folder of brochures from the specialists to hand out or have available. Again, every group member should read the chapter in advance. If you have a guest speaker, jot down any questions you may have before the meeting.

1. What qualities do you think are important in a good listener?
2. What do you think it takes to have as much compassion for oneself as for others? Do you think it is difficult for caregivers to permit themselves to be gentler and kinder toward themselves? Why or why not? Take some time to journal about this. After the journaling exercise, share your insights with the group if you feel comfortable doing so.
3. If you are meeting as a group, consider inviting a professional to your meeting who specializes in veterinary issues and compassion fatigue. Ask the professional to discuss their work and approach to helping with compassion fatigue. Can they recommend some general strategies for self-care?

Note to group leader: to prepare for the next session, each group member should read the next chapter and try one new self-care strategy suggested in the chapter. It may be in any category (emotional and mental, physical, or spiritual).

18

Coping

The Importance of Self-Care

Meditate. Live purely; be quiet; do your work with mastery; like the moon, come out from behind the clouds! Shine.

—THOMAS BYROM'S RENDERING OF THE DHAMMAPADA

If you have read up to this point and think you already have compassion fatigue, you probably do. Don't worry. There is hope, and you have already accomplished the first step on the road to recovery—identifying the problem. You may have already taken some other initial steps to recovery, such as beginning your search for a specialist who can help.

Your next step involves learning how to take care of yourself. This chapter aims to help you increase the behaviors that improve your emotional resilience. You will also be helped greatly by learning ways of caring for yourself physically, emotionally, mentally, and spiritually on a proactive basis. This includes learning how to replenish and nurture yourself daily. Changing habits is difficult, and you may need help to start taking care of yourself. But you can do it! Please don't put it off: take one step today in the right direction.

Being proactive is the key because if we wait for fatigue to happen and the symptoms have already begun to manifest, it is already too late. Veterinary professionals must be adequately prepared to deal emotionally with the care of dying and traumatized pets and their families. The more prepared you are, the less stress you will encounter.

Caring for Yourself Mentally and Emotionally

Helping animals through their illnesses, injuries, and even their deaths is an amazing privilege. Clients need your compassionate care when they are suffering from fear and grief. To respect that privilege, you need to take care of yourself. You cannot provide pets and clients with the best possible care if you are emotionally and mentally depleted.

There are many different ways to take care of yourself mentally and emotionally. We explore some of the main methods in the following sections. Please choose an area to start with today, and then add methods over the next few weeks until they are routine. All these methods work in conjunction with grief and loss or compassion fatigue support; in fact, if you are beginning to see a specialist, they will most likely also focus on helping you learn and implement similar strategies.

Resting and Playing

Has anyone ever asked you questions such as "Can't you ever just sit still and watch an entire movie without having to get up and do something?" If you feel you must always be doing "something," you may have a hard time just resting. Rest is important because it replenishes you.

You may not even realize you are not getting enough rest. Admittedly, it can be challenging to make time for relaxation. After all, there's the laundry to do, pets to feed, people to feed, dishes to wash, plants to water, bills to pay, litterboxes to clean, towels to fold, drawers to organize, and emails and text messages to answer. You do them on automatic pilot, thinking that you are having a day off, but in reality, you are not getting a break at all! These things may be mindless, but they are not restful. If you have a bad case, you may even bring your work home and work extra hours.

If this sounds familiar, you need to teach yourself to let go and relax. It sounds easy, but trust me, the simplest things can be extremely difficult to do if they are new to you. Keep in mind that it is a work in progress. Caregivers typically have a very difficult time even with the mere idea of taking care of themselves. When I suggest that clients begin putting themselves first, they almost always respond as if I were speaking a foreign language!

According to the American Veterinary Medical Association (AVMA), "One of the biggest favors any veterinarian can do for his or her patients, colleagues, and family, is to take selfcare and stress control seriously" (2004). Learn how to stop taking your work home if you haven't already. If you've forgotten how to play, take some lessons from the animals and children you know and relearn how to play. Playing is highly therapeutic, whether it's catch, hide-and-seek, or musical chairs. Get out a board game, play Twister, or just allow yourself to be silly. Let yourself get fully absorbed in whatever you choose to do, just as animals and children do.

Veterinary professionals must find a way to slow down their lives to face the high demands of their profession. We all need time to rejuvenate through proper rest.

Strategies for Relaxation

If you are always "busy," you need to learn how to rest and play. Here are some things you can do when you are feeling overwhelmed:

- Surround yourself with kindhearted, nurturing people.
- Take a hot bath by candlelight.
- Read uplifting literature or a novel just for pure fun.
- Visualize yourself feeling peaceful, calm, and fulfilled, and hold on to those feelings.
- Maintain a nutritious diet.
- Write in a journal.
- Listen to relaxing music.
- Dance around the house while listening to music, or get out the bongos and play along.
- Take five relaxation breaths or practice alternate-nostril breathing (called *nadi shodhana* in yoga).
- Take a walk in nature.
- Center yourself daily, even for just ten minutes at a time. Allow yourself to become fully present. Focus on your life right now, at this particular moment, and not on what happened in the past or what may or may not happen in the future.
- Working your way down, stretch each muscle group while paying attention to your breathing.
- Take time for self-reflection (see textbox "Self-Reflection Techniques" for more information).

Self-Reflection

According to physician and author Dr. Deepak Chopra, it is only through self-reflection that you can truly heal (Chopra and Tanzi 2018). By learning to quiet your mind and witness your own thought process, you can gain the insight necessary to allow change to take place in your life. In one interview, he said, "Pay attention to yourself outside the realm of your experiences, and you'll discover that there is a light there, there is a love there. Love of one, love of all, merge into love, pure and simple. It radiates from you like light from the sun. This love is not sentiment, but the truth at the heart of all creation" (Leach 2016).

Chopra, originally from India, also cited a Vedic saying that "all your life you've paid attention to your experiences, but never to yourself" (Leach 2016). This is something for those of us in the animal-care professions to keep in mind as we manage the symptoms of compassion fatigue. Self-reflection may be difficult at first, and it may even get worse before it gets better. But hang in there—getting back in touch with your true self will sustain you throughout your lifetime.

Taking a Vacation

I am also rejuvenated by spending time in spiritual places like Sedona, Arizona; Santa Fe, New Mexico; and Montecito, California. But if I don't have time to get away and know I need the feeling of doing so, I drive out to the Self-Realization Fellowship's Lake Shrine, just north of the beach on Sunset Boulevard in the Pacific Palisades of California. There I find a tranquil lake surrounded by a Gandhi memorial, meditation gardens, walking paths, and a multitude of friendly ducks, and I am recharged. My suggestion is that you find something similar that restores your balance when needed. Vacations are great, but when you cannot get away for one, you can recharge with a minivacation.

An actual vacation, however, does help you relax more fully unless it is so busy that you come back more stressed than you were when you left. It can also give you a new perspective on your life and something to look forward to. The anticipation of a vacation can be just as valuable as the vacation itself. A couple I know who are both gifted surgeons handle the trauma, stress, and strain of their careers by traveling somewhere incredible at least a couple of times a year. They are entirely devoted to their practices and work long hours, but they schedule their vacations in advance, giving them both something to look forward to and a way to rebalance.

I know one board-certified veterinary oncologist who prefers what I refer to as "remote control therapy." With his physically and emotionally

Self-Reflection Techniques

One exercise in self-reflection comes from Carol A. Lampman, founder and director of Integration Concepts. It includes the use of breath coupled with a list of questions.

Lampman developed the self-examination provided below to help people gain insight into themselves and a new way of looking at the future. Complete these exercises at separate times when you will not be disturbed. You will need a pen and paper to take notes.

Lampman asks that before beginning, the participant take a few minutes to sit while relaxing the body and quieting the mind. Start by breathing deeply and slowing your breath, seeing whether you can fill your lungs "all the way up to your collar bone," if possible. Continue breathing this way for about ten minutes, and then go to the list of questions.

"Try not to 'think,'" Lampman says, "but be open and receptive to any insights that might come. Write down whatever you are aware of without analyzing or questioning. [Analysis] can be done later, along with any additional exploration that might be required for the question." The questions are as follows:

Step One

Self-Reflection Questions

GENERAL

- Are there any integrity issues that need to be cleared?
- Return borrowed items, repay loans, clear up disagreements, etc.
- What do I need to create order in my life?
- Clean house, organize office, clear out closets, fix broken items, etc.
- Am I satisfied with my growth/progress in my work or vocation?

GROWTH

- Am I still holding on to repetitive patterns that no longer serve me?
- Why? What are the secondary gains?
- Am I taking full responsibility for creating my life as I want it to be?
- Is there any place where I am not honest with myself or others?
- Do I blame others or life for my lack or shortcomings?

PERSONAL

- Am I taking care of my body and my health?
- Do I have access to all my emotions and express them productively?
- Are my relationships healthy and satisfying?
- Is there someone (including myself) that I need to forgive?

SPIRITUAL

- Am I willing to let go of control and trust in the highest good for myself or others?
- Am I addressing my spiritual growth and development?
- Am I making time for my spiritual needs and practices?

Step Two

Future Possibilities Questions

PREPARING FOR THE FUTURE: LET YOUR IMAGINATION GO

- What do I want to create more of in the future?
- What activities feed my heart and soul?
- What activities or projects fuel my passion for life?
- What needs to change to create time for these activities?

SEEING THE FUTURE: LET YOUR IMAGINATION GO

For these questions, consider the following as part of the exploration: work, relationship, health, other.

- What does my ideal life look like in the future?
- With this in mind, how do I see myself living one year in the future?
- How do I see myself living five years from now?
- How do I see myself living ten years from now?
- What beliefs might be blocking my ability to create this reality?
- What needs to change, or what do I need to do to create this future reality?
- What positive statement(s) would counteract any negative beliefs and create the changes needed to move forward?
- Am I willing to take the steps and use the tools to change my life?

There is one more question to ask at this point. Is this desire important enough for me to apply the time and effort in order to create this reality? If the answer is yes, you are on your way. If the answer is no or questionable, then further exploration is needed. If you don't know where you are going, you'll get nowhere. A good way to check your desires is to ask yourself, "What is the experience I am looking for?" The answer to this question may expose a longing or yearning for something deeper and far more significant. "It is time to let go of the past and look into the future, creating on the inner realm that which we desire to bring forth into the physical world."

demanding career, he escapes into the television every chance he gets. Maybe surprisingly, this seems to work for him. I don't think it matters what he is watching, only that he is watching. But be careful about trying to relax by watching TV. If you are hypersensitive, the violence and unkindness you see on TV can also be distressing.

Breaking Down Tasks

From the feedback I have received over the years, I've found that one of the most valuable tools recommended for trauma, grief, and compassion fatigue is to break your day or your tasks down into smaller increments of time or portions. This technique can help, especially if you feel so overwhelmed that you cannot face the day (see textbox "Case Study: Lynn").

When you are overwhelmed by life, waking up and looking at the entire day ahead of you can result in feelings of anxiety, sadness, depression, and even paralysis. In such situations, you must learn to break it down.

Here is an exercise you can try right now. Find a pen or pencil and something to write on, and write out all the tasks you need to accomplish today. Remember to include only those things you absolutely must do, not what you think you should do. Next, look through those tasks and number them in order of importance. Take a look at the first item on your list (the one you thought was most important), and break that down as well.

So, for example, if I were feeling overwhelmed by compassion fatigue, but I knew that one of the most important things I had to do that day was get the

Case Study | Lynn

Lynn, a veterinary technician at a busy specialty practice, told me she had gotten to the point where she couldn't get herself out of bed. Overwhelmed by unresolved grief and trauma and the unending battles at work, she woke up every day thinking about the problems ahead of her. She had no idea how to rid herself of this pervasive sense of doom. One day, she just stayed in bed. That day turned into four, and she consequently lost her job. Yet another valuable team member was lost to fatigue.

This crisis point could have been avoided if Lynn had been doing preventive self-care. Breaking her day into segments might have helped.

laundry done (or I would have nothing to wear to work the next day), I would write down all the steps for doing this seemingly menial task. I would then tell myself that all I had to do that day was the first step, gathering up the laundry. Once I gathered it, I would go back to my list and make a check mark by the first step, "Gather the laundry." Making that check mark feels great. It begins the process of bringing up your self-esteem and makes you feel as if you have accomplished something. If I can do that, I would likely feel as if I could then handle making the trip to the washing machine with the dirty laundry (step two). Either I will do that and feel that much better, or I will not—and that's fine, too, because I have given myself permission to do nothing more at that moment than gather the laundry.

Now, for those who are wondering, I am well aware that most people sort their laundry after they have gathered it but before taking it to the washing machine. Not so in my family. With as many children as I have, they are lucky to get their laundry washed at all, and over the years, they have learned that sometimes white underwear turns pink unless they sort it themselves. I advise that if they don't want to do their own laundry, then they will have to learn to like pink. It's one of my boundaries!

Now, back to the subject at hand. When I was ready and feeling up for it, I would put the laundry in the machine, pour in the soap, turn it on, and thereby get to put another checkmark on my list! You can see how this is going. The machine completes its cycle, and I can then tell myself that all I have to do is take out the items and separate the pieces I'll hang up from the pieces that will go in the dryer. At some point, I will actually hang those pieces and start the dryer. Ultimately, I'll take them out of the dryer and fold them. In our house, everyone's clean laundry goes on the island counter in the middle of our kitchen, and everyone is responsible for putting their own laundry away. That's yet another boundary!

By the time I get to that point, I have accumulated so many check marks that my self-esteem has been elevated even more. I no longer have the thought "I still have to do the laundry" looming over my head. Even though I have permitted myself to do only one step at a time, the momentum usually takes over, often resulting in my being able to accomplish far more than I expected, thereby making me feel better about myself and elevating my mood even more.

As we know from previous chapters, our ability to stay on task is typically compromised when we are in the midst of grief or compassion fatigue. When it's paperwork that I have to deal with, particularly things such as paying bills, I find that covering up everything except the particular bill I am working on

Reframing the Problem

When having a particularly difficult time, along with breaking your tasks down, ask yourself what is causing you the most stress at that moment and what is preventing you from doing what you want or need to do. Next, consider looking at ways you might change the problem, accept it, or get away from it altogether. Or perhaps there are ways you can reframe the problem or respond to it differently.

helps immensely with my ability to stay focused and on task. If it's a report that I have to read, I will take a blank piece of white computer paper and tear it in half or fold it so I can cover up all the print after the line I am reading. When we are not ourselves because of loss, trauma, or compassion fatigue, it is easy to become overwhelmed by any and all sensory stimuli. By using these simple methods, you will be able to cut out any excess visual distractions from your work field. Sometimes the simplest things elude us but are of the greatest benefit (see textbox "Reframing the Problem").

Be Easy on Yourself

It is imperative that you learn to be compassionate with yourself, especially when you feel you have failed. Failing or being imperfect is human and a part of everyone's life. You will find your emotional balance much sooner if you don't suppress or exaggerate your disappointments in yourself and if you can accept your failures with kindness. Being mindful is being nonjudgmental and staying open to your thoughts and feelings without trying to deny or suppress them. Honor yourself and know that the more you feel compassion for yourself, the more room you will have to feel compassion for others.

Consider developing your sense of self around who you are, not what you do, and working toward truly knowing that you can't help each and every pet exactly as you would like. Even during difficult times, remember what your own personal gifts are.

Discover which of your beliefs or thoughts might be contributing to your feeling out of balance. Remember, there is no room for self-judgment in grief, trauma, or compassion fatigue. Just as you wouldn't judge others for their pain, you must not judge yourself. When you are feeling beat up by life, concentrate on your wins, on the animals you have helped, not on the ones you haven't (see textbox "A Change of Focus"). Replace negative thoughts with positive ones. This is called cognitive replacement. You must be clear about your own issues and how they may be affecting your work. Cognitive replacement helps stop obsessive thoughts and the tendency to judge yourself harshly; at the same time, it can serve to remind you of your strengths.

One of the most important habits to change immediately is negative self-talk. When you notice that you are putting yourself down, follow it up with a positive self-message. For example, I noticed myself thinking, "I'm absolutely useless, I've been in the veterinary field for eighteen years, and I couldn't even save my own dog. What good am I?" I would then have to force myself to say a positive self-message, such as "Given the resources I had available, along with the knowledge I had of the situation, I made the best decisions possible at every moment, always having my loved one's best interest in mind as my primary concern and motivation."

If positive self-talk is ineffective, try negative reinforcement to use the subconscious mind to avoid unwanted thoughts or behaviors. One professional

A Change of Focus

To stay balanced, you must accept that you have limitations—you are only human! After my first full day of volunteering at the orphanage in Calcutta, Mother Teresa walked me to the gate to say goodbye. I was filled with such joy and a deep sense of fulfillment until the gates opened slightly, and there stood at least fifty more children from the streets, arms outstretched, begging for money.

Distraught, I turned back to look at Mother Teresa and asked, "How do you ever feel like you've done enough?" "No, no, no," she replied. "You have it wrong. You must look at the ones you did help and know that by helping just one, you have helped many, for one life touches another, which then touches another, and it goes on."

Concentrate on what you can do, not on what you can't. Find the things in your life that make you feel powerful, in control, nurtured, and balanced, and regularly bring them into your life. Think of the animals you have been able to help rather than those you couldn't help. No matter how much you do or how much you know, you can't save them all. You can help one animal or one person at a time, and in so doing, you will help change the world.

whose beloved border collie had died implemented this technique. I suggested he keep a rubber band on his wrist and flick it every time he went back to blaming himself for losing his girl. He reported that it was the only thing that was able to shock him into not being consumed by his thoughts of the trauma or beating himself up emotionally. He was thereby able to continue living his own life, which he had seriously considered ending.

Don't forget that accepting that you have been suffering from compassion fatigue only validates that you care deeply about other living beings. Give yourself credit for being such a compassionate individual. Above all, treat yourself with the dignity, respect, and compassion you deserve and accept yourself and your feelings, whatever they happen to be at any particular moment.

Examine Your Coping Mechanisms

Stress is a part of life, and we all learn to cope with it in different ways. Those ways are called coping mechanisms. Some coping mechanisms are healthy and help you find your sense of balance. Others are not so healthy; in fact, some are destructive. All of us, especially caregivers, need to find the things, the people, or the places that de-stress us, and we need to do it proactively, not waiting until symptoms occur. These coping mechanisms, of course, must be healthy.

Detrimental coping strategies include things such as excessive consumption of alcohol, abuse of drugs, and overeating. Spending all your energy helping pets and their people while failing to monitor your own well-being is also a poor coping mechanism, even if everyone keeps saying how wonderful you are for doing it. At some point, it will get to you; it is unsustainable. Staying overbusy can be a way of suppressing your feelings; it can also be a sign that you are judging yourself excessively.

Instead, consider one of the many healthy coping mechanisms suggested elsewhere in this chapter. Whether it's meditation, physical activity, rest, or any other suggestions offered here, try to replace the unhealthy coping mechanisms you may be using with healthy ones.

Setting Limits

Over the years, I have heard several veterinary professionals say that they relate to pets better than they relate to people. This is often because of specific issues they dealt with while growing up. In a subconscious attempt to regain the power they felt they had lost during their childhood, many of these

Thinking About Limits

If you struggle with setting limits, ask yourself the following questions when determining whether a boundary needs to be set:

- Would you feel comfortable asking someone else to do the same thing?
- Would you agree to do this particular thing if you knew that no one would be disappointed or upset with you regardless of your answer?
- Think of someone you know who has good boundaries. How would that person handle this situation?

Remember, everyone has their own comfort level regarding boundaries. Thinking about these questions can help you become more aware of your own current limits and the limits you would like to set.

professionals will have absolutely no limits when it comes to trying to help, save, or heal a pet. They often extend this attitude to the pet's family as well.

Setting healthy boundaries is vital to your well-being and battle against compassion fatigue. If you find that you constantly obsess over the pets you treat, even while not at work, then you could use some limits in your life. To do that, you must realize that no matter how much you do or how well you do it, you cannot help or save all the animals. Choose to focus on the ones you can help. Boundaries are essential to our survival as caregivers and create a sense of safety.

Recognize that you are part of a caregiving team for every pet you work with, and accept that no one can do this work alone. By realizing this, you will better serve the pets, your clients, and yourself, and you will not be as likely to have the negative thoughts known to contribute to compassion fatigue. People who are caregivers by nature and profession tend to give endlessly to others but typically struggle to give to themselves. If we don't learn how to take care of ourselves—and set limits—there will be nothing left to give (see textbox "Thinking About Limits").

Take Care When Making Big Decisions

Compassion fatigue can impair your cognitive abilities, making it more likely that you will make poor choices or choices you will later regret. If you are in the throes of compassion fatigue, I strongly suggest you avoid making any life decisions involving major changes unless and until you have fully recovered. These types of changes could include the decision to marry, divorce, or move in with your significant other; the decision to have more children (two-legged or four); the decision to move to a new home; the decision to quit your job or accept a new one; or the decision to spend an extravagant amount of money. The chance that you will make a decision you will regret is too great, so please, put any major decisions on hold until you find yourself again.

Deal with Your Guilt

To prevent or recover from compassion fatigue, you must permit yourself to take care of your own needs. Sometimes when we do not give ourselves this permission—the permission to provide ourselves with the authentic, sustainable self-care we deserve—the reluctance can be a result of guilt and shame we have not let go of. There are steps you can take to deal with guilt and shame in a positive way. Caregivers who take these steps may find that they can then allow themselves to do whatever is necessary to nurture themselves and heal.

Guilt and shame are often considered synonyms; in reality, they are not the same. Guilt is the feeling that you have done something wrong. It is meant to make you aware of something and implement a change. Shame, however, is the feeling that something is wrong with you—it is about self-punishing.

Feelings of guilt are so common in caregivers that there is actually a recognized phenomenon called "caregiver guilt." The causes of guilt are many and varied. When things don't go as we want them to with our patients, we can feel as though we didn't do the right thing. Or we may blame ourselves or feel we have let our patients and clients down. We feel guilty when we don't live up to our self-imposed expectations, which are often unrealistic to begin with.

Many people hold on to guilt, believing it will keep them from making the same mistake again. But it is only by letting go of the guilt that we can allow true healing to begin. Guilt is not meant to punish; it is intended to motivate us to heal, improve, or correct a situation. But when we are suffering from compassion fatigue, it is difficult for us to see that and use our guilt to move toward corrective behavior. When combined with compassion fatigue, guilt can instead do the opposite: it can become one more thing that immobilizes us both emotionally and physically.

One veterinary professional confessed to me that she was afraid to let go of her guilt because punishing herself every day provided her with a connection to the pit bull she loved and had lost. She was afraid that if she let go of her guilt, that connection would die too. Guilt is a toxic emotion if we allow it to flourish within us. To cope with guilt, we need to recognize and identify it, which is true of any negative emotion. Next, we must be clear about where we feel that we have failed, and then we must examine our expectations.

If we find that our expectations are not realistic, our next task becomes working on letting them go. If they appear realistic, we can then decide how we will act differently the next time those feelings come up.

See the textboxes "Conquering Guilt and Shame" and "Cognitive Restructuring Worksheet" for more information. For the "Cognitive Restructuring Worksheet," the goal is to change "hot thoughts" (e.g., guilt) into more logical, balanced thoughts. First, identify the situation that has brought up feelings of

Conquering Guilt and Shame

Guilt is a part of life, and it is undoubtedly a part of the experiences of trauma, grief, and compassion fatigue. Here are some things that might help you deal with your guilt:

- Know that guilt is a normal and natural reaction to loss, but it is a feeling, and feelings are not to be judged.
- Look at your feelings as they come up for you and label them if you can (e.g., "I'm overwhelmed with feelings of guilt.").
- Assess what triggers that response (e.g., "I shouldn't have put him through that last ultrasound. I wasn't going to do anything invasive anyway because of his age and the condition of his heart, so I should have just let him enjoy the last few days of his life rather than dragging him through yet another procedure.").
- Reframe it (e.g., "I now realize that I would have felt guilty no matter what I did because if I hadn't done the ultrasound, I would have beat myself up emotionally, thinking that if I had just done that last ultrasound, we would have had a better idea of what was going on inside him and may have been able to extend his life.").

There's no "winning" with trauma, grief, or compassion fatigue—you can always find something to feel guilty about—but I assure you that working through the feeling rather than fighting it will help you move more quickly toward healing.

guilt. Next, describe your mood, the thoughts you are having, and the images that accompany these thoughts and feelings. What is the evidence supporting these thoughts and feelings? What is the evidence that does not support them or that contradicts them? List some alternative, more balanced thoughts about the situation. Finally, write down how these more balanced thoughts make you feel.

Feeling Your Feelings

It's very important to understand and give yourself permission to not be okay. Not feeling the need to act or be different from what you truly are or what you are truly feeling is being congruent, and that is the goal. You are entitled to feel afraid, guilty, sad, disappointed, traumatized, depressed, anxious, angry, and lonely from time to time, just like everybody else. More importantly, you are entitled to express such feelings, and you must express them to truly be okay. The key is not to ignore the pain but to recognize it, refrain from judging it, and thereby allow it to move through you. Suffering only increases if we try to hide our pain, if we ignore it, or if we try to fight it.

In our battle against compassion fatigue, most of us need to look at the losses and traumas from our past that we have not yet dealt with (see textbox "Case Study: Dan"). As part of this process, you may also have to work on letting

Case Study | Dan

Dan, a veterinary caregiver, told me his father had died by suicide. This happened when Dan was very young, and consequently, he had never been able to come to terms with the idea of euthanasia. He chose to work with animals, he said, because he wanted to treat them differently; he would never "abandon" them as his father had "abandoned" him.

This wonderful professional felt a great need to save every animal, just as he wished he could have saved his father. But he could not, and as a result he felt powerless. Once he discovered the connection between his father's death and his feelings of inadequacy, he could work on it and eventually let it go.

Think about whether your choices and actions are an attempt to regain the power you felt you lost when you were a child. If you can, talk to a professional to work through these feelings.

go of self-doubt, anger, and fear. You may be suppressing these emotions in an effort to accomplish the goals you have created for yourself. Get back in touch with who you are, what you want, and how you feel.

Start to honor yourself and your feelings and accept that you are human. Things don't always go as we want them to, and you will experience losses, trauma, frustrations, disappointments, and so on, just as we all do. When you react emotionally to these things, it only means that you are human. The more open you are to yourself and to what you are experiencing in the moment, the more compassion you will be able to feel for yourself and, as a result, for all other living beings.

Journaling

Journals can be an excellent way to work through feelings. If journaling is helpful to you, do it frequently. If you have not used a journal in this way before, try the following exercise: Please take a moment to make a list in your journal of all the people you have ever admired and note what you appreciated about them. Then write about how you could bring one or two of those qualities into your life as you reconstruct yourself.

Once you have started writing in your journal, you will be able to think of many similar ways to use it. Later on, you can reread those entries to find strength and encouragement, see how far you have come, and remind yourself of techniques that worked for you.

Staying in the Moment

One skill I use regularly is the Buddhist practice of staying in the moment. When we are in the moment, we are far more likely to be able to handle life emotionally, physically, mentally, and spiritually than if we are dwelling on the past or contemplating and being anxious about the future.

One method of staying in the moment is to keep a daily journal in which you record one thought and one feeling every night just before you go to sleep. You don't have to expound on it, but you can if you desire. For example, a journal entry for one night could be as simple as "I felt incredibly sad today" or "I thought that this just isn't worth it." Or it could be as elaborate as "When I woke up this morning and realized that it was the eighteenth, I was overcome by a deep sense of sadness that lasted the entire day. I thought and can't believe that an entire month has gone by since I lost the love of my life. I missed him so

Cognitive Restructuring Worksheet

Our self-messages can dictate our moods. This worksheet helps you challenge your negative thinking and rescript it for a more positive result or reaction. Fill out this worksheet whenever you feel that your thoughts have been irrational.

What do you view as the event that triggered or activated a response?
(Who? What? Where?)

What mood, emotions, or feelings did you have during the event?

What were your thoughts or beliefs during the event?

What objective evidence do you have to support your view?

What evidence do you have that contradicts your thoughts or beliefs?

Is there a possibility that you are experiencing faulty reasoning?

Are you personalizing?

Did you jump to conclusions?

Are you allowing "shoulds" to dictate your thoughts or behaviors?

Are you "catastrophizing"?

Are you blaming?

What are some alternative and balanced thoughts that you now have about what happened?

What actions can you take to influence the situation or avoid a similar event in the future?

Observe your present mood. What are your emotions and feelings now?

It takes time to learn how to disregard your negative and irrational thoughts and replace them with more adaptive ones. At some point, however, you will be able to do this automatically without even writing it down.

Adapted from Rape Crisis Information Pathfinder, "Looking at Things in a Better Light: Cognitive Restructuring Worksheet," n.d., www.ibiblio.org/rcip/cognitivews.html, which is based on information from Mind Tools Corporation, www.mindtools.com.

much today that I couldn't do anything. I just stayed in bed all day and couldn't even bring myself to brush my teeth, and at times it even hurt to breathe."

When you know you have to make a journal entry of one thought and one feeling every night, your subconscious mind starts to check in with you throughout the day to have something to record that night. This brings you to your goal of being in the moment. Like anything else, the more you do it, the more natural it becomes.

When clients have difficulty accessing those thoughts or feelings, I ask them to notice their surroundings as they sit before me. You can try this, too. I ask them to pay attention to where they are and what is around them, and I ask them to describe what they see and hear. I also ask that they close their eyes and begin to notice what they are sitting on, what their body is touching, and how it feels. "Is it soft and comforting?" I might ask. "Is it scratchy, stiff, hard, or somewhere in between?"

Suppose a client is very analytical by nature and has an even more difficult time accessing their creative or imaginative side. In that case, I ask them to name six things they see in the room and six things they feel (e.g., their arm on the arm of the chair and how the fabric feels underneath, their lower back pressed against the back of the chair, the heaviness in their chest, the stiffness in their neck, their feet on the floor), and three things they hear at the moment (e.g., the sound of my voice, the nature sounds on a compact disk playing softly in the background, birds chirping in the trees, the gardener mowing the grass outside, the hum of the water fountain outside my office window). I then ask the client to identify one smell they are aware of in the moment (i.e., the scent of incense or candles burning, the smell of cats or dogs in the room, or the smell of freshly cut grass).

We are trying to create new habits, and in time, if we stick with things such as staying in the moment and remaining present, we will be better for it. Our sense of balance will not be as easily threatened.

Guided Imagery

Guided imagery, also referred to as guided relaxation, can be used in many ways to help those with compassion fatigue. A compassion fatigue expert may use guided relaxation to help you rediscover what gives you a deep sense of joy, nurturance, fulfillment, peace, or contentment. Here is an exercise you can try on your own or with a partner. (After one of you has completed the exercise, the other person can try it.)

Close your eyes and relax for a few minutes. Just be in the present moment, as described above, until you feel centered. Then, picture yourself in a place that creates in you any or all of the feelings listed in the previous paragraph. Look around you. What do you see? Look to the left and then to the right. What images stand out the most? What colors do you see? What sounds do you hear? Because you are describing something you see in your mind, it could be anything: a natural landscape, a cityscape, or a place you know or knew in your past. Notice every detail. If you have a partner, describe it out loud.

What are you feeling physically? Are you lying down, leaning against something, sitting, or standing? What does that feel like? What colors, sounds, sights, smells, animals, or people are in your special place? Use all your senses and describe them aloud if you are working with a partner.

Once you have found this place, you can re-create it whenever you want to. You might try "going" there for at least five to ten minutes daily. You can always do more, but don't overwhelm yourself at first. Start with a minimal amount of time every day. Even in our busy world, we can all find five or ten minutes daily to do something directed toward our emotional and mental well-being. You can do this type of guided imagery almost anywhere or at any time (but not while driving!). The results will be immediate: your heart rate and pulse rate will decrease as you give yourself fully to being in your own

Quick Fix

How to Decompress

When you are having a particularly stressful day or have had to deal with an emotionally difficult case, find a place where you can go and be alone for five to fifteen minutes to disengage. Sometimes the only place you can be alone in a busy practice is in your car or a bathroom stall. It doesn't matter where it is; what matters is that you find someplace where you can be alone. Once there, you can do some deep relaxation breathing, engage in healing imagery, meditate, or, again, just be.

These are ways to get you through the moment when you are overwhelmed. Deep relaxation breathing involves breathing in through your nose for a slow count of five, holding your breath for another slow count of five, and releasing your breath gently and slowly through your mouth to another slow count of five. Repeat this five times.

special, safe place. You will come back refreshed (see textbox "Quick Fix: How to Decompress" for an exercise that can help even during a busy workday).

Because it relies on primitive brain function, guided imagery is particularly effective in dealing with trauma, grief, and compassion fatigue. Trauma is a biophysical syndrome. Positron emission tomography scans reveal oxygen loss to the neocortex and a "lighting up" of the amygdala during the reintroduction of a trauma. Guided imagery is a form of daydreaming but can be directed specifically for healing and growth. Ideally, it involves all the senses. The body does not discriminate between what is real and what is imagined. Thus, imagery helps reduce anxiety and depression, speed healing, and reduce fear.

Guided imagery also produces a state of relaxation that aids us in accessing the subconscious mind, where buried emotions are stored. This place of healing can bring to the surface painful and traumatic issues that need to be resolved. Through imagery, you can use the power of your own mind to create healing images and focus your energy in positive and self-compassionate ways. In *Dr. Andrew Weil's Mindbody Toolkit* (2006), Dr. Weil states that when talking about guided imagery,

> what we are really talking about is drawing on the power of imagination, which I think is an incredible engine that is part of the elaborate connections of interactivity of the mind and body. Of the many methods available for mindbody treatment, I find that guided imagery is one of the most creative, interesting, dynamic, productive, successful approaches available to patients and physicians.

Progressive Muscle Relaxation

Another technique I have been teaching and practicing for several years is called progressive muscle relaxation (PMR). PMR is very effective in reducing anxiety. It works through alternate tensing and relaxing of various muscle groups throughout the body.

Because of the correlation between stress and muscle tension, you can reduce stress-related symptoms by learning how to relax your muscles. You can practice PMR while sitting or while lying down at night before falling asleep.

Start by closing your eyes and concentrating on feeling your feet. Now tense them for ten seconds and then relax them for twenty seconds. Now, in sequential order, do the same thing with your ankles, calves, thighs, groin, abdomen, chest, shoulders, upper arms, forearms, hands, fingers, neck, ears, jaw, mouth,

Visualization Exercises

Here are three additional visualization exercises you may find helpful:

- Visualize a bubble of protection that surrounds you or a semipermeable wall that allows in only positive feelings and keeps out negative ones.
- Visualize building a wall block by block around your negative emotions and memories.
- Imagine yourself encased in a dome of white light. Loving and protective energy surrounds you from the top of your head to the bottom of your feet, allowing only good and positive energy in, while protecting you from anything dark and negative.

cheeks, forehead, and skull. If you aren't yet noticing how relaxed you are, you are probably asleep! (See the textbox "Visualization Exercises" for more ideas.)

Use of Humor

Try to find the humor in life. Even amid all the pain, humor can exist in the most unlikely places. Animals can be funny; puppies and kittens are particularly so. Even words can be funny, especially when we trip over them or they seem to appear out of nowhere! Like yoga, meditation, or creative outlets, laughter can be very therapeutic and healing.

Although I always recommend being extremely careful about what you watch on television or at the movies, something funny or lighthearted can help create the balance you seek and shield you from further negative stimuli. There are many funny shows. If you are lucky enough to have funny friends, spend time with them. Invite them over for dinner if you must! They will help you see the humorous side of life. The funny thing is that laughing, in and of itself, can lighten your mood.

Benefits of Crying

Interestingly enough, crying is also good for our health. According to Asmir Gračanin, Lauren Bylsma, and Ad Vingerhoets (2014), this notion is supported by scientific research. They stated that researchers consistently find stress hormones in tears. As Dr. Kevin Keough pointed out, stress hormones are known to damage bodily systems, making this connection a critical finding (Cohen and Sherman 2014). Crying is an important biological function and a healthy way to release harmful stress hormones, whether from grief, trauma, loss, or simple sadness and loneliness. It is an excellent coping mechanism for preventing or helping with compassion fatigue.

Creative Outlets

How do you access and use your creative side? If you don't know, then it may be time to find out. It might be through listening to music or playing a musical instrument, gardening, writing poetry, singing, dancing, sculpting, painting, drawing, knitting or sewing, cooking, or doing any other activity that takes creativity. Use any or all of them to help you find your balance. Don't worry about being perfect: if you love to sing but know you are off-key, then go ahead and sing. You're not trying to perform for anyone—the goal is to enjoy it.

Here are some ways to use creativity to express your feelings:

- **Writing:** Writing letters to the pets or people with whom you have unfinished business can be very powerful and healing. You must write just as if you were sending the letter to the recipient, but the value of writing it will come whether you send it or not. Some people bring their letters to an individual or group session or just to a special place and read them aloud. Some keep their special letters in a safe and meaningful place, whereas others choose to burn them after reading them aloud, allowing the breeze to carry the ashes away. Keeping a journal can also be very healing and therapeutic, as described previously.
- **Releasing:** As in the item above, write a letter to a person or an animal. Then fold the note up and put it inside a balloon that is then filled with helium. Next, go to a special spot, a meaningful place that holds special memories, and release the balloon. Watch as it soars upward until the vastness of the sky above finally swallows it. One veterinary technician who did this described the experience as the closest she had felt to her dog since his passing six months earlier. She said, "I know that sending her that message in the balloon somehow

just furthered our connection." Another veterinary caregiver implements this on every birthday or significant anniversary after the tragic loss of her cat, who passed more than three years ago. She adds her own meaningful touch to the ceremony by bringing along some of her cat's favorite snacks and leaving them by a big tree for other animals to enjoy after she leaves. (For other releasing techniques, see the textbox "Releasing Your Worries, Literally.")

- **Dancing and movement:** Expressing your feelings through your body is very powerful, and some professionals specialize in just that. Not that you need to pay someone to benefit from movement and dance! Simply turn on a favorite song and allow your body to express your feelings.
- **Drawing and painting:** Take a pen or brush and allow yourself to create whatever comes to you. Let it flow through you, and let your creations help you heal.

Releasing Your Worries, Literally

Often it isn't easy to let go of intense emotions. The idea of releasing a balloon in which you have put a letter is described in the accompanying text. Here are some other releasing exercises:

- In sand at the beach, write a few words identifying what you are in despair about or what overwhelms or hurts you, and then stand back and watch as the water takes it away.
- Write out your sorrow and mindfully walk over to a trash can and symbolically toss it in, with the idea that once it is in the garbage, you are released from the weight of having to carry it with you.
- Write out your painful feelings and experiences on a small piece of paper and symbolically burn it or drop it in a "worry box" or "healing box" that you create. You can dump all your worries into the garbage on the last day of every month.
- Take a warm, nurturing bath, which in and of itself is healing, but when you are finished, imagine your pain, grief, anxiety, anger, or frustration washing down the drain.

Caring for Yourself Spiritually

Research has shown that a sense of spirituality and faith can facilitate the healing process. One study reported lower blood pressure, less time spent in hospitals, and fewer strokes in those who considered themselves religious than in those who didn't participate in any particular spiritual activities (Koenig 2004). This study also noted that elderly people who either meditated or prayed had longer lives on average than those who did not.

Another study revealed that spirituality can change your brain structure (Newberg 2010). This research, which involved brain imaging, showed that when Buddhists meditated or nuns prayed, their frontal lobes were active. This area of the brain controls language and attention. This means spiritual practices can help us remain connected and at our best when dealing with pets and their families. It therefore doesn't matter what your beliefs are—the positive effects on the brain are identical regardless of the religion or spiritual practice adhered to. Newberg also revealed that, like a muscle that is being conditioned, the frontal lobes can grow thicker over time.

Other research has shown that people with a sense of spirituality seem to find the strength needed to fight life's challenges more easily than those without this sense. This includes finding the strength to battle diseases, cope with traumatic events, and recover from crises with an increased sense of strength. It seems that feeling a connection to something larger than ourselves plays an essential protective role in our lives.

If you already have spiritual beliefs, go ahead and pursue them. They're good for you. If you feel you do not relate to spiritual things, you can still benefit from practices that are traditionally considered "spiritual." It's possible to meditate without having a religious focus. (See textbox "Meditation Basics" for tips on beginning a meditation practice.)

Meditation

Meditating gives me a sense of calm, balance, and healing. It recharges me so I can be at my best for those who come before me, be they two-legged or four.

Just about everyone can benefit from meditation. What's more, some forms of prayer (contemplative or centering prayer) are similar and can be just as beneficial as meditation. Whether you take a class or read a book to learn how to meditate, do try integrating it into your busy lifestyle (see textbox "Meditation Basics" for tips on beginning a meditation practice). You will be surprised how quickly it will help. (See also the above section "Caring for Yourself Spiritually.")

Meditation Basics

Starting a meditation practice will give you a sense of calm and peace that will help you significantly in the battle against compassion fatigue. Meditation can benefit anyone coping with anxiety and stress. Meditation provides the practitioner with a break from the world—from work, cell phones, the Internet, and all the other demands of our lives. As our lives become more and more suffused with technology, the solitude and silence of meditation become more critical than ever.

There are many ways to meditate, and no one method is better than another. Try different styles and use what works for you. To begin, wear comfortable clothing and sit or lie down in a comfortable position. Try to keep your back as straight as possible and close your eyes. You can meditate anytime and anyplace, but try to choose a peaceful environment, especially at first. Some people like to create an altar of some sort to sit before. This altar may display items that are meaningful to you or give you a sense of connection. You may choose to dim the lighting and use a candle to create a relaxing atmosphere.

Many people like to meditate in silence; others enjoy listening to meditation music or the sounds of nature. YouTube has many videos with music chosen to accompany a meditation session. You can also listen to the sounds of nature, either via a recording or, if you are in an area with sounds that comfort you, by simply opening the windows. There are even "recordings" of silent meditation timers ending with a pleasant gong sound to let you know that your twenty minutes are up. You can find them online by typing "meditation timers" into your search engine.

Many people choose to recite a mantra while meditating. A mantra is a word or phrase used to protect the mind from wandering. When I was nineteen, I was taught the Hong-Sau method of breathing, which involves breathing in to the word *hong* and breathing out to the word *sau* during meditation. *Hong* and *sau* are ancient Sanskrit words that can be extremely calming. But the word you use does not have to be prescribed by anyone. You can choose any word or phrase that resonates with you, or you may choose to observe and follow your own breath, as calming the breath tends to calm the mind simultaneously.

Some people prefer to return to a calming image instead of a mantra or the breath when their minds begin to wander. You may find comfort in focusing on the mental image of a candle, a flower, a lotus, Buddha or Christ, or any symbol that centers your spirit. As mentioned earlier, some people like to do a guided form of meditation. Guided imagery can speed healing and growth while using the imagination to move toward a conscious goal. Unguided, silent meditation has a slightly different focus—to let go of thoughts and sit in calm awareness. The purpose of the mantra, image, or focus on the breath is to help you return to this intention.

If your mind begins to wander while trying to meditate, simply and gently remind yourself of this intention by returning to your breath, mantra, or image. If your technique uses attention to breath, the point is not to control the breath but to observe it, thereby calming your respiration and simultaneously decreasing both your pulse and your blood pressure.

To use the breathing technique, begin by simply feeling your breath as it comes into your lungs; as it departs, allow yourself to relax. Rest your tongue gently against your teeth at the roof of your mouth. Exhale fully and focus on pushing out all the air in your lungs. Now slowly fill your lungs back up by breathing in through your nose to a count of eight; to relax more fully, hold your breath to a count of seven, and then exhale through your mouth for another count of eight. This is often referred to as the *relaxation breath*.

The benefits of this type of breathing are many. The parasympathetic system is strengthened even when the technique is used during day-to-day traumatic or stressful situations you may encounter. Breathing this way will allow you to regain your balance quickly and can help build a strong connection between your mind and body.

I recommend the following resources to anyone interested in learning more about meditation:

- *Insight Meditation: A Step-by-Step Course on How to Meditate*, by Sharon Salzberg and Joseph Goldstein (Sounds True, 2002).
- *The Most Direct Means to Eternal Bliss*, by Michael Langford (Freedom Religion Press, 2008).
- *Breathe! You Are Alive: The Sutra on the Full Awareness of Breathing*, by Thich Nhat Hanh (Educa Books/Full Circle, 2008).

Caring for Yourself Physically

Taking care of yourself physically, mentally, emotionally, and spiritually will help you find the fastest route to healing. It will also help you prevent compassion fatigue. The three most significant physical components of self-care are diet, exercise, and simply getting a good night's sleep.

In the battle against compassion fatigue, it's crucial to become aware of what you are consuming. When you suffer from compassion fatigue, it's easy to reach for the wrong things. You may try to comfort yourself by grabbing cookies, chocolate, or ice cream, but as you know, these things are very transitory, and they end up making you feel worse than you did before.

Instead, determine to eat a healthy diet. You can even choose foods that will target your emotions and truly make you feel better. Foods that contain tryptophan, an essential amino acid, are natural mood elevators. They are known to relieve depression and stimulate the production of serotonin, a neurotransmitter in the brain that regulates sleep, appetite, and emotions. Tryptophan can be found in fish, lentils, turkey, chicken, beans, carbohydrates, zinc, folic acid, and certain vitamins.

I also recommend a diet rich in superfoods, which, because of their high vitamin and mineral content (including trace minerals), are known to prevent some types of cancer and provide us with energy and vitality. According to Dr. Steven Pratt, superfoods "contain high concentrations of crucial nutrients . . . [that] have been proven to help prevent and, in some cases, reverse the well-known effects of aging, including cardiovascular disease, type II diabetes, hypertension, and certain cancers" (as cited in Pratt 2023; Pratt and Matthews 2006, 2013). Blueberries, for instance, are filled with antioxidants and protect against heart disease and premature aging. Kale, another superfood, has many antioxidants and may, along with other leafy green vegetables, reduce the risk of cancer and help slow the aging process. Please be aware that this information is not intended as medical advice, and I suggest you consult your primary care physician before making any major changes in your diet.

Other plant-based superfoods for you to consider include avocado, beans, broccoli, garlic, nuts, onions, tea, and wild salmon (Pratt 2023).

Keep in mind that many natural supplements can help alleviate stress. Some of the most common ones that might benefit you are listed below. However, check with your primary care physician before taking any of these supplements, especially if you have any health issues or are taking any medications.

5-HTP	Has been known to help with stress and depression.
Rhodiola	A Siberian herb that many say fights fatigue and depression.
Melatonin	Chronic stress, a component of compassion fatigue, can deplete this hormone, and low melatonin levels are linked with anxiety and sleep disturbances.
Lactium	A milk-based protein that is said to promote relaxation.
Eleuthero	A Siberian herb known to boost stamina and immunity while reducing fatigue.
B vitamins	Essential to energy production and nerve function.

In addition, get those endorphins flowing by exercising. Get your heart rate up, and you will have administered a dose of your own personal antidepressant. A gifted veterinary surgeon with whom I have worked maintains his inner balance as a triathlete. Others do yoga or aerobics, hike, or join a cross-fit gym. Experiment until you find an exercise program you love. Most experts agree that exercising a minimum of thirty minutes, three days a week is important to staying healthy. It strengthens the immune system, reduces stress, elevates mood, and maintains a healthy heart.

Most of the time, taking care of yourself is common sense. You already know these things; you just may not be doing them. To fight compassion fatigue, you have to do them. So when you are tired, rest. If you are thirsty, drink some water. If you are hungry, nourish yourself. Each week, make time for exercise.

In addition, engage in hobbies outside your profession. This can give you something to look forward to, as well as a sense of accomplishment. Maybe it's taking care of a bonsai garden. Maybe it's making jewelry, cooking, writing poetry or music, doing photography and creating scrapbooks, visiting vintage shops or swap meets, or making pottery. If you've neglected yourself for so long that you have no hobbies, start to think about what you could do that would be pleasurable and help you de-stress. When you do the things you love, you are nurturing yourself and ensuring you don't fall prey to compassion fatigue. Discover your joy!

I attended a seminar titled "Coping with Compassion Fatigue in the Animal Care Community," presented by the Humane Society University, in which they discussed tools to identify the importance of balance in one's life. I have found some of these tools to be enormously helpful, such as the Wheel of

Life from the book *Co-Active Coaching: Changing Business, Transforming Lives* (Kimsey-House et al. 2018).

You now have a toolbox filled with many self-care tools, each designed to prevent compassion fatigue and put compassion-fatigued veterinary caregivers on the road to recovery. Get to know these tools by working with them. Share them with other members of your team. When everyone on the veterinary practice team uses self-care strategies, everyone benefits, including patients and clients. Each team member will find greater fulfillment on the job. The practice will become a healthier workplace, one filled with positive, enthusiastic people who find great satisfaction in caring for others, are authentic and compassionate, and are ready to meet the challenges of the day.

For the Trainer

To prepare for this session, each team member should have already read this chapter and tried at least one new self-care strategy. Discuss the following:

1. Many different self-care strategies are suggested in this chapter, and group members were assigned to try one new strategy during the week. Which strategy (or strategies) did you try? Did you find this helpful? Why or why not? Share your experiences if you feel comfortable doing so.
2. Are there other strategies you have tried on your own that you found helpful over the years? If so, please share these ideas; other group members may be able to benefit from them.

19

Creating a Personalized Self-Care Plan

Self-compassion is the first step toward compassion for others.

—THE DALAI LAMA

Now it's time to create your self-care plan. This is a personalized plan designed just for you. Take out a blank piece of paper and divide it into five sections. Label them as follows: Spiritual, Physical, Emotional, Cognitive, and Support System (SPECS). You can think of your SPECS as your specifications for where you want to be in your life, what you want to attain—or you can think of them as your "spectacles," your way of seeing yourself and your life clearly.

First, identify what your goals are in each of these areas. What do you want to accomplish, both short and long term? Next, write down specific steps you will take to attain each of those goals. Below, I provide some questions to get you started. You may want to write in your journal first for each area, taking up as much space as you want, and then decide what will go on your final list.

Spiritual

What makes your spirit soar? What inspires you? What makes you feel connected? What rejuvenates you? What gives you a sense of balance, calm, and peacefulness? Identify these things and write them down. Are there things that work against you spiritually that you want to avoid? Write these down, too. Next, identify your spiritual goals. How will you attain them? Give yourself specific, doable short- and long-term goals.

Physical

What are your physical outlets? What physical activities do you do to take care of your body? What do you do physically that calms you, makes you feel good about yourself, or gives you a sense of your own physical power? Identify these and record them. What goals do you have for your physical self, and how can you reach those goals? Write down specific ways to achieve them.

Emotional

What makes you feel happy and safe? What gives you joy? What places make you feel good? What animals? What people? What do they look, sound, smell, or feel like? Write down those things that lead to positive emotions for you. What goals do you have for your emotional self? How can you attain these goals? Again, be specific.

Cognitive

Throughout the book, we've been calling this taking care of yourself "mentally." This area focuses on conscious thoughts rather than emotions. What thoughts inspire and empower you and make you want to be your best? Where do those thoughts typically come from? What thoughts allow you not to judge or blame yourself but rather to accept yourself just as you are? What goals do you have for how you think about things, for how you think about yourself? How can you succeed in attaining these goals?

Support System

Make a list of the people on whom you can depend. Who constitutes your social support system? How can you use their support for your success in attaining the goals you have set in your self-care plan?

Those who make it onto this list will be those closest to you and whom you have known for a long time. They have earned your trust and vice versa. You have come through for them on many occasions, and they have done the same for you. Although you do not want to burden your friends and family

How to Run a Debriefing Session

Debriefing sessions allow veterinary professionals to reflect on what they have experienced while caring for particular animals and clients. Debriefing should be offered at least once a week and can also be used on an as-needed basis. The facilitator should help participants focus on their emotional responses to any losses or traumatic experiences, the grief they may be experiencing, and the relationships they have shared with others during these experiences.

After everyone is welcomed to the debriefing session, introductions are made, if necessary, and the purpose of the debriefing is reviewed. Those in attendance are then asked to begin by describing their relationship to the pet or their involvement in the pet's care. The particular circumstances at the time of the loss or trauma are discussed next. I try to ask only open-ended questions so that those who are sharing will feel comfortable describing the experience from their perspective. For example, the facilitator may ask questions such as "What was the most difficult part of taking care of this patient?" "What was the most satisfying part?" "What was it like to take care of this pet?" "What have your experiences been like since the trauma (or loss) occurred?" "What did working with this pet teach you?" Once the feelings are expressed, the facilitator can help normalize them for the caregiver as part of the process of recovery from trauma or loss, lead a discussion of coping strategies that may be applicable, and remind participants of available support resources. The facilitator can also make referrals as needed.

with your grief on a regular basis (as described in chapter 18), sometimes you will need someone to lean on who is willing to listen to you. Everyone needs this from time to time, and you can reciprocate by doing the same for those with whom you have your closest relationships.

People who support each other like this don't need to spill out their emotions all the time. Sometimes they can offer support by being together. Maybe you have a friend who has been through thick and thin with you, and you've enjoyed many a walk in the park or lunch out together. You've confided in each other about countless things. She should be on the list. Or maybe it's your brother who lives in another state, but you know you are there for him, and he's there for you. Again, put him on the list. It could be a mentor who helped you get through veterinary school or your aunt who is like a second mother. Write down their names.

If your support system is light, it may be because you haven't had time for anyone lately. That's not surprising—it's how you got to where you are now amid a battle with compassion fatigue! Try to reconnect with people who are important to you to build your support system. In the meantime, try setting up what I call "debriefing sessions." I recommend this to all the veterinary practices I work with. These sessions should be scheduled regularly (see textbox "How to Run a Debriefing Session"). Knowing that you have a regular place to go where you can talk about all the difficult emotions you are carrying is a real asset in fighting compassion fatigue. I also suggest having a professional on staff to whom team members can turn as difficult feelings arise.

Maintaining Healthy Habits

It is important not only to start new good habits, but to make them last. As a caregiver, one of the challenges I've had in maintaining my own self-care is practicing what I preach. It is a work in progress for me, as it will be for you. To ensure that you stay on track, try the following techniques:

- Make a "pact" with a colleague or friend who also wishes to use self-care strategies. Check in with each other regularly to stay accountable.
- Experiment with different self-care strategies until you find the ones that work best for you. Some of the suggestions in this book will appeal to you, and others will not. The key is to find the ones that click.
- Figure out ways to turn your favorite self-care strategies into habits. A wealth of recent research has shown the effectiveness of this concept. For aid in developing this idea, see *The Power of Habit: Why We Do What We Do in Life and Business* by Charles Duhigg (2014).

Once you find self-care strategies that work for you, you will find you look forward to doing them. Doing these activities regularly and proactively will enable you to avoid being swallowed up by the very work that gives your life meaning and fulfillment.

Remember, preventing compassion fatigue, or recovering from it once you have it, will be an ongoing process. It requires your continual attention. If something in your plan isn't working, revise the plan. Being proactive is the key. As you know by now, if you wait until you have compassion fatigue before you do anything about it, it's already too late! The pets you treat and their people need you, and they are fortunate to have you. But to continue to be there for them, you must first protect yourself.

Recommended Resources

The Green Cross Academy of Traumatology, which offers help to traumatized people and animals worldwide, has compiled "Standards of Self Care Guidelines" (https://greencross.org/about-gc/standards-of-care-guidelines/). These guidelines can be beneficial to any caregiver in creating a self-care plan. They are very detailed and are based on the premise that caregivers must use self-care strategies to ensure high-quality care to others. The academy believes "it is unethical *not* to attend to your self care as a practitioner because sufficient self care prevents harming those we serve." It is well worth reading the entire set of guidelines.

Another good resource is the Compassion Fatigue Awareness Project (https://compassionfatigue.org). This site includes three excellent charts: "The Ten Laws Governing Healthy Change," "The Ten Laws Governing Authentic, Sustainable Self Care," and "The Ten Laws Governing Healthy Caregiving." These charts may motivate you and help you follow through with your self-care plan.

For the Trainer

By the time of this session, participants should have read the chapter and be well on their way to completing their SPECS: the worksheet on their Spiritual, Physical, Emotional, Cognitive, and Support System. Discuss the following:

1. Go through each of the five sections of the SPECS worksheet. Share some of your most important goals and how you expect to reach them. If the group is large, consider splitting into pairs to discuss the SPECS. For each of the five sections, the pairs can change so that each person will get to share with five other participants. The facilitator may use a clock or watch to time the segments. Some of these pairs may wish to become "accountability partners" in the future, as suggested above under "Maintaining Healthy Habits."
2. After this SPECS review, discuss the following: Did any of you learn more from your colleagues' answers than you expected? How might you change your own list based on these additional insights? Use what you learned to revise your list this week.

20

Now Where?

The Future of Compassion Fatigue in the Veterinary Industry

You must be the change you wish to see in the world.

—MAHATMA GANDHI

Compassion Fatigue Among Staff

Compassion fatigue causes organizations to go through increased turnover rates, workers' compensation costs, absenteeism, and employee stress. It is possible to heal an organization plagued by compassion fatigue, but it can take a long time. The remedy must start at the top. When those in administrative positions become aware of the detrimental effects of compassion fatigue on employees, they must act. Better yet, they should be proactive and institute preventive measures before a problem arises.

The preventive and remedial measures must follow through the ranks and reach all team members. Compassion fatigue can be eliminated through awareness, respect, and proactive care and concern. Proper orientation and training, coupled with ongoing support, can ensure a competent and emotionally healthy staff.

When I talk to new veterinary interns and others who have recently finished veterinary school, I am always amazed to learn that there are still programs that have no training in place for teaching the importance of understanding the human-animal bond, of knowing how to handle the delicate issues of grief and loss, or of learning how to prevent compassion fatigue. All universities and veterinary schools must begin an early intervention approach, teaching the importance of proactive self-care in all veterinary professions. This is vital to ensuring that we, as a profession, stop losing good people to something that could have been prevented.

To train their graduates to provide the best possible care to patients and clients, veterinary schools, residencies, and technician programs must be more effective in covering what to expect from clients, conflict management, grief, communication skills, stress management, and proactive self-care. Just as veterinary care team members must be sources of ongoing support for their patients and clients, they must also support their own efforts and continued emotional well-being.

Healthy Workplace

Supportive work environments must be provided to veterinary professionals, with a place to debrief from difficult cases and a place to receive the emotional support necessary for continued care. Such places can be provided on-site or off-site—it doesn't really matter as long as it is nearby.

"The Ten Laws Governing a Healthy Workplace," developed in 2003 and revised in 2013 by the Compassion Fatigue Awareness Project (compassionfatigue.org), are simple yet informative and helpful. The list sets forth ten rules that specify employer responsibilities. For example, rule 1 says, "Employer provides debriefing for staff following any traumatic event." Rule 6 states, "Employers provide positive team-building opportunities to promote strong relationships among colleagues." Other rules specify that employers provide "continuing education for staff" and promote good communication skills. The veterinary profession should adopt similar rules to ensure a healthy workplace.

In addition, it would be enormously helpful to administer psychological testing as one of the criteria for veterinary school admission. Many times, veterinary caregivers realize that they are not well suited for a career in veterinary medicine only after going through veterinary school and spending several miserable years in practice. The challenges of continual trauma and loss and compassion fatigue finally get to them, but it isn't easy to switch gears and begin a new career. They have made a considerable financial investment, may still owe on their student loans, and have suffered emotional consequences that will take time to heal.

Financial Support

Dr. Robert Larner of the Robert Larner, M.D. College of Medicine at the University of Vermont provided a model based on the field of human medicine that we can follow in veterinary medicine (2024). Dr. Larner was responsible for creating a culture of giving back throughout the alumni community, and along with his own compassionate and generous nature, he created thousands of MDs who could graduate from medical school and were ensured a medical education second to none, and this extended to generations of future physicians as well.

May the large, corporate veterinary medical groups follow the lead of Merck Animal Health, which provides $5,000 scholarships to second- and third-year students in accredited veterinary schools (AVMF 2022), and the Humane Society Veterinary Medical Association (HSVMA), which gave five veterinary students $10,000 scholarships in 2023 (Schrader 2023). Corporate practices throughout North America can seize the opportunity to help veterinary medicine mitigate compassion fatigue by offering full scholarships, which would also impact veterinary student attrition and debt.

Remember, as tuition costs continue to rise at veterinary medical colleges and universities, so too does the financial burden on most graduating veterinarians. As the 2020 AVMA Graduating Senior Survey showed, the debt typically incurred by graduating veterinarians was approximately $157,146 (Mattson 2020, citing Bain 2020). This factor is considered a prominent driver of the elevated suicide rates within the veterinary profession.

The 2023 AVMA Graduating Senior Survey noted that the "mean debt-to-income ratio . . . fell a third straight year to 1.3 times the amount of a graduating veterinarian's income" (Nolen 2023b, citing Doherty 2023). Although it is a decline, it is still significant debt. A National Public Radio interview with epidemiologist Suzanne Tomasi noted that student loan debt is still a factor in veterinary suicide (Spidel 2023).

As a compassion fatigue specialist, I have worked with hundreds of interns at several veterinary specialty hospitals. The internship year they spent with us could be considered grueling. It was not uncommon to hear that they were exhausted, hungry, and often scared to death that they wouldn't be able to endure and would possibly have to drop out of their internship programs. Over the years, several confessed to me that even if they could make it through the internship, they were highly concerned about the debt they would soon have to repay.

I never went to the specialty hospitals without bringing food for the interns and other staff members. The fear and exhaustion, coupled with the lack of nutrition, need to stop because, as several told me, they couldn't afford groceries.

In addition to offering scholarships, large veterinary corporations could also proactively sponsor the cost of mental health resources for those experiencing compassion fatigue. As a veterinary support specialist, I found that those practices that offered mental health resources for compassion fatigue lowered their rates of employee absenteeism as they increased their rates of company loyalty.

Grief Support Programs

I also believe that university grief support lines, usually staffed by students, should be redesigned as more helpful tools with professional, well-trained staff. The support lines have often been known to do more harm than good with the current arrangement. One woman who later became my client told me about her experience with one of these support lines. When she called a grief support line offered by a highly respected veterinary school, the person who answered the phone put her on hold after the caller revealed that she had thoughts of harming herself—definitely not a good thing to do to someone who is suicidal! The client said the only reason she didn't hang up the phone that day and end her life was that she became curious about how long she would be expected to wait. The grief support "professional" did not return for a full seven minutes! Fortunately, in this case, the client was so surprised that she went from thinking about suicide to anger at the support line's incompetence. The experience motivated her to call the number someone had given her the previous week—my number. We need further training for those who can find themselves holding a human life in their hands by virtue of what they do.

Through pre–veterinary school psychological testing, a decrease in veterinary school debt, supportive work environments, proactive self-care, continuous clinical training, and on-site or off-site grief and compassion fatigue support, veterinary professionals would be better able to meet their professional responsibilities without sacrificing themselves.

The AVMA's "Workplace Wellbeing 1: Setting the Foundation" program (2025b) indicates that veterinary community members should be in position to protect their health and well-being through five modules, including the following:

1. A New Era for Wellbeing at Work
2. How to Request, Receive, and Give Feedback Effectively
3. The Intersection of Workplace Conflict and Wellbeing
4. QPR Suicide Prevention Training
5. Diversity and Inclusion

The AVMA now defines compassion fatigue and acknowledges the pain it entails by citing the ProQOL tool (2025a). It is encouraging that the AVMA has taken notice. It is a start. Moreover, the American Animal Hospital Association (AAHA) has taken a leadership role in increasing awareness, not only by publishing the first edition of this book but also by publishing others that focus on related issues (some of which can be found in the reference list). The word may spread, and awareness may increase. You can become part of the solution now that you have read this book. Begin with your own self-care program, and then tell your colleagues. Pass the book along and use the "For the Trainer" sections. You will be doing your peers a favor.

Proactive Practice

Your own clinic or hospital need not wait for the entire profession to catch up with you. As a veterinary team, you can work on this together. If you do, I believe that the morale at your practice will be high. You will develop a good sense of team collaboration. Peer support, job satisfaction, and a sense of belonging to an efficient team will increase.

To be proactive as a practice, you will need to encourage effective and open communications, teach coping skills, honor the need for time off, provide community outreach programs and in-services, offer informal activities outside work, provide positive new staff orientations, and offer ongoing emotional support through group and individual consultations. What are your goals as a practice, and how will you achieve them? Devise a plan and a multipronged approach to ensure your team members get the support they need.

In this book, I sometimes use the metaphor of a journey. We discuss taking first steps, and I note that the journey is for the long haul. If your practice decides to institute a plan that involves everyone working on these things together, no one will have to walk the road alone.

Good luck with your journey. I hope this book helps you along the way.

Acknowledgments

I am thankful for Madelyn Weston, assistant project editor at Texas A&M University Press. I greatly appreciate her kind guidance throughout this entire process.

I want to thank Nathan Davidson, executive acquisitions editor at Rowman & Littlefield Publishing. I continue to respect his expertise, his deep kindness and his compassion.

Marj Atkinson's knowledge as a librarian was extremely helpful in helping me in fact-checking this updated edition.

I am appreciative of Kelley Robbins, associate acquisitions editor at TAMU Press, for her dedication and her deep commitment to excellence.

I want to acknowledge and am grateful for my assistant, Trevor Curran, and his assistance in bringing this edition to completion.

Glossary

assertive communication: A style of communication in which individuals express their thoughts, feelings, and needs clearly and directly while respecting others' rights and boundaries.

avoidance behaviors: Actions taken to escape or prevent exposure to situations, thoughts, or feelings that cause anxiety or discomfort.

behaviorist: A mental health professional who focuses on observable behaviors rather than internal mental states, emphasizing the role of environmental factors in shaping behavior.

body language: A type of nonverbal communication in which physical behaviors, as opposed to words, are used to express or convey information, such as being at the same physical level as a client, uncrossing arms, eye contact, and so forth.

burnout: A condition that occurs when, in responding to excessive stresses and demands, individuals demand too much of themselves, eventually becoming overwhelmed, exhausted, apathetic, and negative.

caring-killing paradox: The emotional conflict experienced by veterinary professionals and animal shelter workers who must euthanize animals while also being committed to their care and well-being.

chronic suffering: Persistent physical or emotional pain that continues over an extended period, often affecting quality of life.

cognitive restructuring: A therapeutic technique that involves identifying and challenging negative thought patterns and replacing them with more balanced, realistic ones. Also known as cognitive replacement.

compassion: A heartfelt understanding of the difficult situation of another to the point that one is moved to take action of some sort.

compassion fatigue: Acute emotional pain accompanied by physical, spiritual, and mental exhaustion that stems from caregiving.

compassion fatigue specialist: Someone who listens to those who are traumatized, afraid, grieving, or suffering from compassion fatigue and who understands the veterinary field.

compassion satisfaction: The positive feelings derived from helping others or doing work that contributes to the greater good.

compounded grief: Grief caused by cumulative losses appearing within a short period.

coping mechanism: A behavior that helps people deal with stress or unpleasant emotions.

cyberbullying: The use of electronic communication to intimidate, harass, or harm others, often through social media, text messages, or online platforms.

debriefing session: A group session in which a facilitator helps participants focus on their emotional responses to any losses or traumatic experiences.

decompress: To relax and eliminate nervous tension or anxiety.

denial: Declaring something to be untrue and reacting by engaging in harmful behaviors to avoid the truth.

dissociative reactions: Flashbacks and intense psychological distress when exposed to something that symbolizes an aspect of a traumatic event; can include feelings of detachment and memory loss.

emotional flooding: An overwhelming surge of intense emotions that can temporarily impair one's ability to think clearly or respond rationally. It involves a rapid series of intrusive thoughts and memories of a traumatic event that can cause strong emotional reactions.

emotional triggers: Specific stimuli that cause a strong emotional response, such as anger, sadness, and fear. Triggers can be words, events, memories, people, places, smells, things, and so forth.

empathy: The capacity to see things from another's point of view and feel what that person is feeling.

equanimity: A state of mental balance and composure in the face of challenging situations.

ethically challenging situations (ECS): Situations in which veterinarians face conflicts between professional responsibilities, client wishes, animal welfare, financial constraints, and personal values. These challenges often involve decisions about euthanasia, treatment options, client confidentiality, and balancing the needs of animals, clients, and public health. Veterinarians must navigate these complex situations while upholding their professional ethics and considering the best interests of all parties involved.

ethics fatigue: The mental and emotional exhaustion experienced by professionals when faced with frequent ethical dilemmas or moral challenges in their work.

euthanasia: The practice of intentionally ending a life to relieve suffering, often applied in veterinary medicine for animals with terminal illnesses or severe injuries.

extrovert: A personality type characterized by a tendency to seek stimulation from the external world and enjoy social interactions.

grief: A normal response to loss; a period of intensely painful emotions that begins with the loss of a loved one.

guardian protector: A role or personality type focused on safeguarding and caring for others, often associated with protective instincts and a strong sense of responsibility.

healthy workplace: A supportive work environment including a place to debrief from difficult cases and a place to receive the emotional support necessary for continued care.

highly sensitive person (HSP): An individual who experiences heightened sensitivity to physical, emotional, or social stimuli, and who often processes information more deeply than others.

human-animal bond: The emotional connection and mutually beneficial relationship between humans and animals, often characterized by mutual affection and companionship.

intracardiac euthanasia: A method of euthanasia in which the euthanasia solution is injected directly into the heart, typically used only when intravenous access is impossible.

introvert: A personality type characterized by a tendency to focus on internal thoughts and feelings, often preferring solitude or small group interactions.

journaling: A personal developmental tool that involves writing down your thoughts, feelings, and observations so you can better understand yourself.

learned helplessness: A psychological condition in which individuals believe they have no control over their situation and stop trying to improve or change it, even when opportunities arise.

meditation: A practice that involves techniques to enhance attention and awareness, allowing individuals to detach from automatic, analytical thinking.

mindful communication: Awareness of our thinking and the choices we make in communicating.

mindfulness: A mental state and practice of focusing one's awareness on the present moment, acknowledging and accepting thoughts, feelings, and sensations without judgment.

mirror neurons: Brain cells that activate both when individuals perform an action and when they observe someone else performing the same action, potentially playing a role in empathy and learning.

moral fatigue: The emotional and psychological strain experienced by those who frequently face morally challenging situations or decisions in their work or personal life.

old-school euthanasia: Traditional or outdated methods of euthanasia that may be considered less humane or efficient compared to modern techniques, including bypassing initial sedation.

palliative care: A more holistic and natural approach to end of life care for pets and other animals to help support quality of life and mitigate suffering.

perfectionist: A person who strives for flawlessness and sets extremely high performance standards, often accompanied by critical self-evaluations and concerns about others' opinions.

personal boundaries: The limits and rules individuals set for themselves within relationships, defining the behaviors they will accept from others and those they will not.

pet-owner attachment: The emotional bond between a human and a pet.

physiological reaction: Any physical or psychological reaction to stress, such as headaches, digestive issues, pounding heart, difficulty sleeping and concentrating, pain, anxiety, or fatigue, among others.

post-traumatic stress disorder (PTSD): An anxiety disorder that occurs after one experiences or observes a traumatic event involving significant injury, death, or the threat thereof.

proactive practice: The habit of taking initiative and anticipating potential problems or needs before they arise, often applied in professional or personal development contexts.

Professional Quality of Life Scale (ProQOL): A standardized assessment tool used to measure the positive and negative effects of helping others, particularly in caring professions.

progressive muscle relaxation (PMR): A relaxation technique involving the systematic tensing and relaxing of different muscle groups to reduce stress and promote physical relaxation.

reflective listening: Conveying to clients that the listener values and understands them by reflecting back on what clients say.

reframing: A cognitive technique that involves changing one's perspective on a situation to view it in a more positive or constructive light.

resilience: The ability to adapt, recover, and maintain psychological well-being in the face of adversity, stress, or challenging life events.

secondary stress disorder: A natural, but potentially disruptive, psychological response to learning about or witnessing trauma experienced by others

secondary traumatic stress: A component of compassion fatigue that involves work-related, secondary exposure to extremely stressful events.

self-care: The practice of taking action to preserve or improve one's own health, well-being, and happiness, particularly during periods of stress.

self-compassion: The practice of treating oneself with kindness, understanding, and acceptance, especially in instances of failure, suffering, or inadequacy.

self-reflection: The process of observing and evaluating one's own thoughts, emotions, and behaviors.

social media risk: The risk of incorrect information being shared on social media that can negatively affect the careers of veterinary and animal-care professionals.

stress: The emotional, mental, and/or physical strain that results from too many pressures and demands in one's life, typically from external sources.

sympathy: Similarity or agreement between two or more individuals relating to a viewpoint or emotional response.

therapy animal: An animal used to help people cope with and recover from some physical and mental health conditions.

trauma reminders: Stimuli or situations that trigger memories or emotional responses related to past traumatic experiences.

traumatologist: A mental health professional specializing in the treatment of those who have experienced trauma.

unresolved trauma: Traumatic experiences that have not been properly processed or integrated, potentially leading to ongoing psychological distress or behavioral issues.

veterinary attachment: The strong bond between veterinary professionals and their patients.

veterinary grief: The emotional reaction to the loss of a patient, which can be especially profound when there is a strong attachment to the animal.

veterinary hospice: Supportive and compassionate, quality end-of-life care provided to pets.

veterinary resilience plan: A focus on proactive self-care to prepare for and endure challenging situations inherent in veterinary medicine.

vicarious trauma: The cumulative negative effect of experiencing the trauma of others, to the extent that it can result in dissociation from both professional and personal relationships, as well as intrusive images and nightmares, despair, and resignation.

visualization: A mental technique involving the creation of vivid mental images to achieve specific goals, reduce stress, or enhance performance.

workplace gossip: Any talk about a coworker, whether personal or professional, innocuous or slanderous.

work-related stress: Physical, emotional, or mental strain caused by the pressures and demands of one's job or workplace environment.

References

AAHA (American Animal Hospital Association). 2023. https://www.aaha.org/

Alkema, K., J. M. Linton, and R. Davies. 2008. "A Study of the Relationship Between Self-Care, Compassion Satisfaction, Compassion Fatigue, and Burnout Among Hospice Professionals." *Journal of Social Work in End-of-Life & Palliative Care* 4(2): 101–19.

American Psychiatric Association. 2025. *Diagnostic and Statistical Manual of Mental Disorders* (DSM-5-TR). https://www.psychiatry.org:443/psychiatrists/practice/dsm

Andolina, D., and A. Borreca. 2017. "The Key Role of the Amygdala in Stress." IntechOpen. https://doi.org/10.5772/67826

Aron, E. 1999. *The Highly Sensitive Person's Workbook*. Broadway Books.

Aron, E. 2020. *The Highly Sensitive Person: How to Thrive When the World Overwhelms You*. Kensington Publishing.

AVMA (American Veterinary Medical Association). 2004. "Managing Stress and Avoiding Burnout." https://www.avma.org/javma-news/2004-08-15/managing-stress-and-avoiding-burnout

AVMA (American Veterinary Medical Association). 2020a. "Guidelines for the Euthanasia of Animals." https://www.avma.org/resources-tools/avma-policies/avma-guidelines-euthanasia-animals

AVMA (American Veterinary Medical Association). 2020b. "Veterinary School Admission 101." https://www.avma.org/education/veterinary-school-admission-101.

AVMA (American Veterinary Medical Association). 2025a. "Wellbeing Assessment for Veterinarians." https://myvetlife.avma.org/rising-professional/your-wellbeing/wellbeing-self-assessment

AVMA (American Veterinary Medical Association). 2025b. "Workplace Wellbeing 1: Setting the Foundation." https://axon.avma.org/local/catalog/view/product.php?productid=22

AVMF (American Veterinary Medical Foundation). 2022. "2022 Merck Animal Health Scholarship." https://www.avmf.org/our-impact/education-support/scholarships-and-awards/2022-merck-animal-health-scholarship-2/

Banfield Pet Hospital. "Veterinarians & Superior Petcare." 2023. https://www.banfield.com/

Bartram, D. J., and D. S. Baldwin. 2008. "Veterinary Surgeons and Suicide: Influences, Opportunities and Research Directions." *Veterinary Record* 162(2): 36–40. https://doi.org/10.1136/vr.162.2.36

Bekiari, A., and V. Pachi. 2017. "Insights into Bullying and Verbal Aggressiveness Through Social Network Analysis." *Journal of Computer and Communications* 5(9): 79–101. https://doi.org/10.4236/jcc.2017.59006

Bicknell-Hentges, L., and J. J. Lynch. 2009. "Everything Counselors and Supervisors Need to Know About Treating Trauma." Paper presented at the American Counseling Association Annual Conference and Exposition, March 19–23, 2009, Charlotte, North Carolina. https://manifold.counseling.org/system/resource/4/e/9/4e92f84f-8620-4800-b757-8c1af09c9277/attachment/2e58d100551a9837a38aebde243a8e86.pdf

Bowlby, J. 1969. *Attachment and Loss.* Vol. 1, *Attachment*. Basic Books.

Byrom, T., trans. 1976. *Bhikkhu Vagga of the Pāli Dhammapada (Compilation)*. Shambhala Publications.

Center for Victims of Torture. 2023. https://www.cvt.org/

Chopra, D., and R. E. Tanzi. 2018. *The Healing Self: A Revolutionary New Plan to Supercharge Your Immunity and Stay Well for Life*. Harmony Books.

Cohen, G. L., and D. K. Sherman. 2014. "The Psychology of Change: Self-Affirmation and Social Psychological Intervention." *Annual Review of Psychology* 65:333–71. https://doi.org/10.1146/annurev-psych-010213-115137

Compassion Fatigue Awareness Project. 2010. "What Is Compassion Fatigue?" http://www.compassionfatigue.org/pages/compassionfatigue.html

Compassion Fatigue Awareness Project. 2013a. "The Ten Laws Governing Authentic, Sustainable Self-Care." https://www.compassionfatigue.org/pages/TheTenLawsAuthenticSelfCare.pdf

Compassion Fatigue Awareness Project. 2013b. "The Ten Laws Governing Healthy Caregiving." https://compassionfatigue.org/TheTenLawsHealthyCaregiving.pdf

Compassion Fatigue Awareness Project. 2013c. "The Ten Laws Governing Healthy Change." http://www.compassionfatigue.org/pages/TheTenLawsHealthyChange.pdf

Compassion Fatigue Awareness Project. 2013d. "The Ten Laws Governing a Healthy Workplace." http://www.compassionfatigue.org/pages/TheTenLawsHealthyWorkplace.pdf

Davidson, I. J. 2017. "The Ambivert: A Failed Attempt at a Normal Personality." *Journal of the History of the Behavioral Sciences* 53(4): 313–31. https://doi.org/10.1002/jhbs.21868

Duhigg, Charles. 2014. *The Power of Habit: Why We Do What We Do in Life and Business*. Random House.

Eysenck, H. 1997. *Dimensions of Personality*. Taylor and Francis. https://public.ebookcentral.proquest.com/choice/publicfullrecord.aspx?p=5265438

Figley, C. R. 1995. *Compassion Fatigue: Coping with Secondary Traumatic Stress Disorder in Those Who Treat the Traumatized*. Routledge.

Figley, C., and R. Roop. 2006. *Compassion Fatigue in the Animal-Care Community*. Humane Society Press.

Finkelman, S., Y. Berkowitz, and I. Meir. 1995. *Chofetz Chaim: A Lesson a Day; The Concepts and Laws of Proper Speech Arranged for Daily* Study. 1st ed. Mesorah Publications and Chofetz Chaim Heritage Foundation.

Goetz, M. L., A. Jones-Bitton, J. Hewson, D. Khosa, D. Pearl, D. J. Bakker, S. T. Lyons, and P. D. Conlon. 2020. "An Examination of Myers-Briggs Type Indicator Personality, Gender, and Career Interests of Ontario Veterinary College Students." *Journal of Veterinary Medical Education* 47(4): 430–44. https://doi.org/10.3138/jvme.0418-044r

Goldberg, N. 2009. *The Complete Guide to Women's Health*. Ballantine Books.

Gračanin, A., L. M. Bylsma, and A. J. J. M. Vingerhoets. 2014. "Is Crying a Self-Soothing Behavior?" *Frontiers in Psychology* 5. https://www.frontiersin.org/articles/10.3389/fpsyg.2014.00502

Green Cross Academy of Traumatology. 2023. "Standards of Care." https://greencross.org/about-gc/standards-of-care-guidelines/

Huggard, P., B. Hudnall Stamm, and L. A. Pearlman. 2013. "Physician Stress: Compassion Satisfaction, Compassion Fatigue and Vicarious Traumatization." In *First Do No Self Harm: Understanding and Promoting Physician Stress Resilience*, edited by C. Figley, P. Huggard, and C. Rees. Oxford University Press. https://doi.org/10.1093/acprof:oso/9780195383263.001.0001

Human Animal Bond Association. 2022. "Educate." https://humananimalbond.net/education/

Humanmeterics. 2022. "Discover Your Personality Type." https://www.humanmetrics.com/personality

Hutchison, W. D., K. D. Davis, A. M. Lozano, R. R. Tasker, and J. O. Dostrovsky. 1999. "Pain-Related Neurons in the Human Cingulate Cortex." *Nature Neuroscience* 2(5): 403–5. https://doi.org/10.1038/8065

Integration Concepts. 2023. "Integral Breath Therapy." https://www.integrationconcepts.net/

Jinpa, T. 2015. *A Fearless Heart: How the Courage to Be Compassionate Can Transform Our Lives*. Hudson Street Press.

Keirsey, D. 2022. "Keirsey Temperament Assessment." https://keirsey.com/temperament-overview/

Kimsey-House, H., K. Kimsey-House, P. Sandahl, and L. Whitworth. 2018. *Co-Active Coaching: The Proven Framework for Transformative Conversations at Work and in Life*. 4th ed. https://coactive.com/resources/books/coactive-coaching-4th-edition.php

Koenig, H. G. 2004. "Religion, Spirituality, and Medicine: Research Findings and Implications for Clinical Practice." *Southern Medical Journal* 97(12): 1194–200. https://doi.org/10.1097/01.SMJ.0000146489.21837.CE

Koller, E. C., R. A. Abel, and L. E. Milton. 2022. "Caring for the Caregiver: A Feasibility Study of an Online Program that Addresses Compassion Fatigue, Burnout, and Secondary Trauma." *Open Journal of Occupational Therapy* 10(1): 1–14. https://doi.org/10.15453/2168-6408.1847

Langford, M. 2008. *The Most Direct Means to Eternal Bliss*. Freedom Religion Press.

Larner College of Medicine, University of Vermont. 2024. "Financial Services: Tuition and Financial Aid." https://www.med.uvm.edu/studentservices/financialservices/financialaid/institutional-funding

Lawrence, C. 2009. "Shock Central: Veterinarian Suicides." *Horsemen's Corral*. http://www.corralonline.com/articles/article080310152649.htm

Leach, M. 2016. "We Are the Thinker Behind the Thought." Interview with Dr. Deepak Chopra. Share International Archives. April 29, 2016. https://web.archive.org/web/20160429031039/https://www.share-international.org/archives/religion/rl_mlDeepak_C.htm

Lengyel, K. 2018. "Understanding, Avoiding and Conquering Ethics Exhaustion." DVM 360. July 8, 2018. https://www.dvm360.com/view/understanding-avoiding-and-conquering-ethics-exhaustion

Massachusetts General Hospital. 2018. "'It's All in the Eyes': The Role of the Amygdala in the Experience and Perception of Fear." ScienceDaily. August 21, 2018. https://www.sciencedaily.com/releases/2018/08/180821145223.htm

Mattson, K. 2020. "Veterinary Educational Debt Continues to Rise." JAVMA News. December 3, 2020. https://www.avma.org/javma-news/2020-12-15/veterinary-educational-debt-continues-rise

Meir, I., A. Daina, and C. D. Keller. 2015. *Sefer Chofetz Chaim*. 1st ed. Israel Bookshop Publications.

Myers-Briggs Foundation. 2022. "Myers-Briggs Overview." https://www.myersbriggs.org/my-mbti-personality-type/mbti-basics/

Neff, Kristin. 2015. *Self Compassion: Stop Beating Yourself Up and Leave Insecurity Behind*. Yellow Kite.

Newberg, A. 2010. *Principles of Neurotheology*. Ashgate.

Nhat Hanh, T. 1975. *The Miracle of Mindfulness: An Introduction to the Practice of Meditation*. Beacon Press.

Nhat Hanh, T. 2008. *Breathe! You Are Alive: The Sutra on the Full Awareness of Breathing*. Educa Books/Full Circle.

Nolen, R. S. 2023a. "Updates from the AVMA Feature Resource to Combat Cyberbullying." American Veterinary Medical Association. January 7, 2023. https://www.avma.org/news/updates-avma-feature-resource-combat-cyberbullying

Nolen, R. S. 2023b. "Veterinary Starting Salaries Rise in 2023, Educational Debt Holds Steady." American Veterinary Medical Association. November 1, 2023. https://www.avma.org/news/veterinary-starting-salaries-rise-2023-educational-debt-holds-steady

NOMV (Not One More Vet). 2023. https://www.nomv.org/

Ostaseski, F. 2017. *Five Invitations: What the Living Can Learn from the Dying*. Flatiron Books.

Peale, N. V. 2011. *The Power of Positive Thinking*. Anniversary ed. Ishi Press.

Peng, X., W. K. W. Lau, C. Wang, L. Ning, and R. Zhang. 2020. "Impaired Left Amygdala Resting State Functional Connectivity in Subthreshold Depression Individuals." *Scientific Reports* 10(1): 17207. https://doi.org/10.1038/s41598-020-74166-x

Pet Partners. 2020. "Empirical Support for Therapy Animal Interventions." https://petpartners.org/publications/empirical-support-therapy-animal-interventions/

Pratt, S. G., MD. 2023. "SuperFoods." Super Healthy Living. Archived at https://web.archive.org/web/20230207021130/https://superhealthyliving.com/superfoods/

Pratt, S. G., MD, and K. Matthews. 2006. *SuperFoods HealthStyle*. HarperCollins.

Pratt, S. G., MD, and K. Matthews. 2013. *SuperFoods Rx for Pregnancy*. Wiley.

PsychAlive. 2011. "Dr. Dan Siegel—On Disorganized Attachment in the Making." March 3, 2011. https://www.youtube.com/watch?v=zovtRq4e2E8

Quain, A., S. Mullan, P. D. McGreevy, and M. P. Ward. 2021. "Frequency, Stressfulness and Type of Ethically Challenging Situations Encountered by Veterinary Team Members During the COVID-19 Pandemic." *Frontiers in Veterinary Science* 8: 647108. https://doi.org/10.3389/fvets.2021.647108

Rauvola, R. S., D. M. Vega, and K. N. Lavigne. 2019. "Compassion Fatigue, Secondary Traumatic Stress, and Vicarious Traumatization: A Qualitative Review and Research Agenda." *Occupational Health Science* 3(3): 297–336. https://doi.org/10.1007/s41542-019-00045-1

Reeve, C. L., S. G. Rogelberg, C. Spitzmuller, and N. Digiacomo. 2005. "The Caring-Killing Paradox: Euthanasia-Related Strain Among Animal-Shelter Workers." *Journal of Applied Social Psychology* 35(1): 119–43. https://doi.org/10.1111/j.1559-1816.2005.tb02096.x

Ricard, M. 2012. *Happiness: A Guide to Developing Life's Most Important Skill*. Little, Brown.

Rinpoche, T. S., II. 2015. "Renunciation." In *Teachings from Tibet: Guidance from Great Lamas*, edited by N. Ribush. Lama Yeshe Wisdom Archive.

Saakvitne, K. W., and L. A. Pearlman. 1996. *Transforming the Pain: A Workbook on Vicarious Traumatization*. W. W. Norton.

Salzberg, S., and J. Goldstein. 2002. *Insight Meditation: A Step-by-Step Course on How to Meditate*. Sounds True.

Schrader, H. 2023. "HSVMA Awards 2023 Compassionate Care Scholarships at $10,000 Level: Five Veterinary Students Recognized for Access to Care Efforts." Humane Veterinary Medical Alliance. https://www.humanevma.org/index.php?option=com_content&view=article&id=1348:2023-compassionate-care-scholarship-recipients&catid=23:students&Itemid=93

Schultz, K. 2008. "An Emerging Occupational Threat?" DVM 360. https://www.dvm360.com/view/emerging-occupational-threat

Scott, E. 2023. "Reduce Stress with Increased Assertiveness." Verywell Mind. https://www.verywellmind.com/reduce-stress-with-increased-assertiveness-3144971

Seymour, K. 2000. "Compassion Fatigue/Secondary Trauma." Proceedings of the Annual Convening of Crisis Intervention Personnel, University of Illinois Chicago. Archived at https://web.archive.org/web/20100603201000/http://www.uic.edu/orgs/convening/compassion.htm

Siegel, D. J. 2020. *Developing Mind: How Relationships and the Brain Interact to Shape Who We Are*. 3rd ed. Guilford Publications. https://drdansiegel.com/book/the-developing-mind/

Simpson, L. R., and D. S. Starkey. 2006. "Secondary Traumatic Stress, Compassion Fatigue and Counselor Spirituality: Implications for Counselors Working with Trauma." https://manifold.counseling.org/system/resource/8/c/d/8cd385e4-52c9-4f27-bc35-ea0a4d210d96/attachment/0c10ff43e062adff646a44a5564126b9.pdf

Smith, M. M., S. B. Sherry, S. Chen, D. H. Saklofske, C. Mushquash, G. L. Flett, and P. L. Hewitt. "The Perniciousness of Perfectionism: A Meta-Analytic Review of the Perfectionism-Suicide Relationship." *Journal of Personality* 86, no. 3 (2018): 522–42.

Smith, P. 2009. *To Weep for a Stranger: Compassion Fatigue in Caregiving*. Createspace.

Spidel, A. 2023. "Why Suicide Rates Are High Among Veterinary Professionals." National Public Radio. December 19, 2023. https://www.npr.org/2023/12/19/1220443869/why-suicide-rates-are-high-among-veterinary-professionals

Stamm, B. H. 2010. *ProQOL Manual*. ProQOL. https://proqol.org/proqol-manual

Tomasi, S. E., E. D. Fechter-Leggett, N. T. Edwards, A. D. Reddish, A. E. Crosby, and R. J. Nett. 2019. "Suicide Among Veterinarians in the United States from 1979 Through 2015." *Journal of the American Veterinary Medical Association* 254(1): 104–12. https://doi.org/10.2460/javma.254.1.104

VHA (Veterans Health Administration). 2020. "Passport to Whole Health." US Department of Veterans Affairs. https://www.va.gov/WHOLEHEALTHLIBRARY/passport/

Villalobos, A. 2009. "Quality of Life Scale." Veterinary Practice News. November 30, 2009. https://www.veterinarypracticenews.com/quality-of-life-scale/

Villalobos, A. E. 2011. "Quality of Life to the End of Life: We Owe It to Them!" *Latham Letter*, Spring 2011. Reprinted by San Antonio Humane Society. https://sahumane.org/images/stories/pdf/petcaretips/quality_of_life_to_the_end_of_life_villalobos.pdf

Waeltz, J. 2019. *The Overlooked Side of Compassion Fatigue: Secondary Traumatic Stress* (blog). Dr. Jeni Waeltz. December 17, 2019. https://www.drjeniwaeltz.com/blog/the-overlooked-side-of-compassion-fatigue-secondary-traumatic-stress

Watkins, T. 2010. "Paper Delves into British Veterinarians' High Suicide Risk." CNN. http://www.cnn.com/2010/WORLD/europe/03/26/england.veterinarians.suicide/index.html

Weil, Andrew. 2006. *Dr. Andrew Weil's Mindbody Toolkit*. Sounds True.

Index